Julie,

It's a great time to
be a healthcare marketer!

— Chris Bevolo

EMBRACING THE NEW PARADIGM

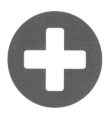

JOE PUBLIC II

EMBRACING THE NEW PARADIGM

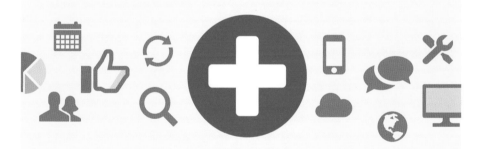

A strategic guide to digital and content marketing
for hospitals and health systems

BY CHRIS BEVOLO
WITH ADAM MEYER

I N T E R V ∧ L

Washington Ave. N., Suite 250, Minneapolis, MN
thinkinterval.com

Printed in the United States of America
First Edition 2011

Published simultaneously in electronic format

Library of Congress Control Number: 2014944866

ISBN: 978-0-9905126-0-8

4

ACKNOWLEDGMENTS

First and foremost, thanks goes to Adam Meyer, principal of interactive strategy and design at Interval. Adam and I have worked together for nearly a decade, and he not only is the source of many of the digital philosophies, perspectives, and issues featured in this book but also is responsible for pushing me and our firm to embrace and master digital marketing. We would not be where we are today without his passion, his business sense, his design sense, and—maybe most importantly—his intellectual curiosity. This book would not exist without Adam, which is why he shares a byline on the cover.

Thanks also goes out to the rest of the Interval crew, most importantly our director of operations and client account manager, Jackie Olson. She's the glue that keeps it all together.

Special thanks to Chris Boyer and Tom Teynor, who played an instrumental role in shaping my thoughts on the new paradigm, whether by encouraging us to push further, teaching me new perspectives, or pushing back hard on wacky ideas or perspectives. The same goes for clients, partners, associates, competitors and friends, listeners of the Arrogant Healthcare Marketing Podcast, presentation attendees, members of the Orlando Party Boat, believers in *Joe Public One*, and all the others who have asked tough questions, shared their stories, and displayed a great sense of humor. The conversations I have shared with healthcare marketers over the past few years have shaped the attitudes and content I share here.

Finally, thanks to my future wife, Tonya, for all of her support and encouragement, and of course to my awesome kids, Jack, Julia, and Callie. I love you all.

ABOUT THE AUTHORS

CHRIS BEVOLO

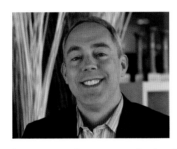

Joe Public II—Embracing the New Paradigm, was written by Chris Bevolo. A nationally recognized futurist, author, and speaker on healthcare marketing, strategy, and branding, Chris helps organizations better understand and leverage key trends in healthcare competition, branding, and consumerism. He is best known for helping healthcare organizations reenvision what their marketing could be, reenergizing management, and inspiring staff to think bigger and act differently. His 2011 book, *Joe Public Doesn't Care About Your Hospital*, a manifesto for transforming healthcare marketing, has become the field guide for driving transformation in hospital marketing departments across the country.

Chris is a frequent keynote speaker and featured presenter at national healthcare conferences on the topics of marketing, branding, innovation, the patient experience, and consumer trends. He has also authored two other books, *A Marketer's Guide to Measuring Results* (2010) and *A Marketer's Guide to Brand Strategy* (2008), as well as numerous articles and papers on healthcare marketing and branding.

Chris founded Interval in 1995, and he and his team have worked with dozens of healthcare clients, including Banner Health (Phoenix, AZ), Providence Health & Services (Seattle, WA), (Falls Church, VA), St. Joseph Health (Orange, CA), Penn State Hershey Medical Center (Hershey, PA), Baptist Health System (San Antonio, TX), Allegiance Health (Jackson, MI), St. Joseph's Hospital (St. Paul, MN), and the Children's Hospitals and Clinics of Minnesota (Minneapolis, MN).

In 2013, Chris founded Blue Lake Brand Consulting, an organization that offers brand guidance to healthcare organizations in transition. Chris serves as a principal at Blue Lake while continuing his leadership role at Interval.

Chris earned an MBA at the University of St. Thomas in Minneapolis and holds a BS in journalism and mass communication from Iowa State University.

ADAM MEYER

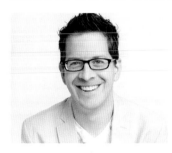

Adam Meyer, principal of interactive strategy and design at Interval, made significant contributions to this book. Adam's background in design, web development, and healthcare marketing gives him the ability to look at marketing challenges from a very broad perspective. He has helped shape the agency's philosophies around interactive strategy, and his passion for evolving and emerging web technologies ensures a forward-thinking approach to client projects. Adam began his career as a game designer for Fanball.com, experiencing firsthand the dot-com boom of the late '90s. He moved from the startup scene to healthcare in 2001 as a designer for North Memorial Healthcare, a Level I Trauma Center in the Twin Cities. Although he came in to work on traditional marketing efforts, he quickly became a conduit for communication between marketing and IT. His role shifted to interactive initiatives, and soon he was leading the design and development of the organization's website and interactive strategies. In 2006, Adam ventured out on his own, running a successful freelance business for two years before joining Interval as creative director in 2008.

It was Adam who prompted Interval to begin its popular healthcare marketing podcast, The Arrogant Healthcare Marketing Bastards. For six years he has helped lead Interval and clients forward, integrating emerging technologies and best practices into interactive marketing strategies. He was instrumental in shaping many of the philosophies outlined in Interval's manifesto for healthcare marketers, *Joe Public Doesn't Care About Your Hospital.*

Having grown up with guitar in hand in his father's radio station, Adam has music and audio engineering in his blood. Adam has worked as a disc jockey and financed his higher education as a professional guitarist and vocalist. To this day, music and audio work remains a passion, with Interval's podcast being just one outlet.

Planning to be an illustrator, Adam began his education as an art major at Minnesota State University, Moorhead, and graduated with a bachelor's degree in marketing management from Concordia University in St. Paul. A variety of programming and database courses taken along the way sparked a passion for the web (which, at the time, was just becoming mainstream), and a melding of these interests helped pave his professional path.

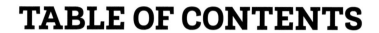

TABLE OF CONTENTS

INTRODUCTION

The two-hour meeting was almost over, and the room was buzzing. The client team had just heard all the ideas—ideas that captured everything we believed mattered, everything that could make a real difference for their marketing efforts. Much of what I had summed up in my 2011 book, *Joe Public Doesn't Care About Your Hospital*, was reflected. The effort would reflect a true transformation in healthcare marketing.

We were going to hit the market in a different way. Not pimping ourselves, beating our chests, bragging about our awesomeness, but rather delivering relevant content about health and wellness that our audiences would value. We weren't going to blow out a million-dollar, billboard-encrusted mass advertising campaign that touted our award-winning-state-of-the-art-cutting-edge whatever. We were going to use a responsive website as the foundation for a digitally based, content-marketing campaign, using SEO, SEM, email, social media, and other effective and efficient tactics to engage our audiences. All of this would be done in a way that would not only reflect the client's brand position but actually help further *build it*. And we were going to measure our progress and results every stinkin' step of the way, in dozens of different ways, to truly understand what was working so we could adjust accordingly. This was a new approach; it was big, it was bold, and most importantly, it would be incredibly effective.

The client marketing team was jazzed. In prior meetings, we had laid out the philosophies, building the foundation for change, and they were enthusiastically on board. Yes, this was different, but that's what they wanted. The principles of digital and content marketing were made clear, and they were excited to see them come to life. Over the last hour and fifty minutes, we had laid it all out, showing them how it would come together.

It was at that point I noticed the vice president of marketing had become quiet. The leader of the group, she had asked smart questions throughout and helped lead the team through some of the issues that had risen, all along championing the new direction. But now she was silent. I looked at her and asked what she was thinking. Her eyes grew wide with realization and, to some extent, terror.

"Holy &%$#," she said. "This is really different. I mean *really* different. And I get it. And you get it. We all get it. But will *they* get it? Those within our organization, will they get it? I mean holy &%$#, how in the hell are we going to sell this? Because this is *soooo* different."

This book is for the client in that meeting and for all the others who agree with the foundational changes in *Joe Public Doesn't Care About Your Hospital*. It's for those who believe that the status quo in hospital and healthcare marketing is ripe for destruction. For those who believe the best way to market our organizations is, in many ways, the polar opposite of the way we've done it for decades and still predominantly do it today. **Most importantly, this book is not just for those who believe these things but for those who want to make change happen.**

MAKING IT REAL

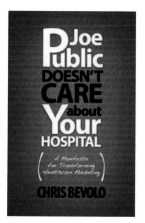

The first "Joe Public" book was a manifesto for change. (From here on, I will refer to the first book as *Joe Public One*. Note that reading *Joe Public One* is not a requirement for moving forward with this book. The brief references used here in the introduction help provide those who *have* read the first book with a clear connection to this one and should provide any necessary context for those who haven't.)

In that book, I laid out five key ways healthcare marketers needed to change to deliver true value to their organizations, and the arguments behind those changes. Those changes, as I defined them in the book, were these:

Change One: Joe Public doesn't care about your hospital

One of the greatest errors of healthcare marketing is the assumption that consumer audiences care about your organization as much as you do. This sin is repeated over and over, in organization after organization, and the prevalence of this problem (and the resulting ineffectiveness) is the reason the book is titled

15

after this change. Without the ability to move past this roadblock, it will be impossible for healthcare organizations to fully embrace the other changes.

Change Two: Out with the old, in with the new

This chapter speaks to the need for healthcare marketers to move beyond traditional methods that are no longer as effective—methods that, unfortunately, are very commonplace in our world. It conveys the attitude you'll need to adopt if you want to break ties with the past and move into a brighter and more successful future.

Change Three: Breaking bad habits

Throughout our industry, many of us are guilty of falling into habits that hamstring our ability to deliver successful marketing. Examples are driving healthcare marketing strategies based on internal pressures ("politically driven" marketing) or always following what others are doing in the market rather than setting our own course ("me-too" marketing). Becoming aware of and then consciously replacing unproductive habits with those proven more effective will help us to become much more successful marketers.

Change Four: Breathing life into zombie brands

Most healthcare leaders have a hard time understanding the definition of branding, let alone working to build their organization's brand in a strategic way. "Zombie brands" are brands that are left to wander the market without guidance or support from their own organizations, and they must be replaced by brands that are actively defined, developed, and managed.

Change Five: Measure, measure, measure

Once we've convinced leadership to let us work in a new way, we must prove that our new approaches to healthcare marketing are actually working. That means we must put into place the structure that will allow us to measure the results of our efforts. From a career perspective, healthcare marketers should consider marketing measurement a "life-or-death" proposition.

In *this* book, I want to focus on those changes that truly fly in the face of how we've always marketed our hospitals and health systems, ways that still dominate healthcare marketing. Furthermore, rather than being a manifesto describing the *what* and *why* of those changes, this book is much more about the *how*. First, let's reconsider the changes outlined in *Joe Public One*.

Two of those changes—the final two chapters related to branding and measurement—didn't represent new or radical ideas. Organizations have pursued branding as a strategic endeavor for 50-plus years. And measuring marketing results certainly isn't a wild-hair idea. In both cases, the problem was that our industry—hospital and health system marketing—was sorely behind other industries in understanding, valuing, and pursuing these disciplines. Advocating for stronger branding and more measurement was on some levels a "duh," but unfortunately it needed to be said (and even more unfortunately, it still does). But in both cases, the ideas of brand and measurement are not contrary to industry beliefs (just industry practice).

In a similar vein, the changes called for in Chapter 3 of the original "Joe Public" book—breaking bad marketing habits—were also, once identified, hard to argue with. Seeking to become a leader rather than a follower by abandoning "Me-Too" marketing? Sticking with a strategic marketing plan to help with "Whack-a-Mole" marketing? Fighting for a seat at the strategic table by practicing "Big M" marketing? Any novelty here came from the fun descriptions; the problems were widely recognized throughout the industry. Other than "Focus Group Fixation," there wasn't much within the bad habits chapter that seemed significantly off the beaten track, hard to understand, or worthy of argument.

That leaves the changes covered in the first two chapters of the book, which really addressed how hospitals and health systems proactively connect with consumers in support of their marketing goals. These changes were different from the others. Chapter 1 of *Joe Public Doesn't Care About Your Hospital* was a call to move away from chest-beating promotional messaging and toward relevant content that provides value in terms of education, health, wellness, and more. Chapter 2, which advocated "Out with the old, in with the new," seems innocuous enough. Who doesn't want to embrace new, improved strategies, tools, and channels to pursue more effective marketing? The problem, of course, is that hospitals not only lag behind other industries in leveraging new strategies, tools, and channels, but they also embrace and prioritize old-school marketing channels and methods. So in both cases, these two chapters called for changes that stood in direct contrast to what the industry did and, for the most part, believed.

LOOK OUT, PARADIGM SHIFT AHEAD

When taken together, these changes in how provider organizations *connect with consumers*—moving away from promotional, mass advertising to digital and content mar-keting—represent a true paradigm shift for the healthcare industry. As with any paradigm shift, the magnitude of change is massive, the resistance strong, and the shift itself years in the making. Marketers are making changes and moving forward, which is all that I hoped for with *Joe Public One*. But the truth is, we're still not moving fast enough. That's not a total surprise because, as I stated earlier, this is truly a *paradigm shift*, which implies a completely different way of thinking or approaching a particular set of beliefs based on a funda-mental shift in assumptions. Moving from the Ptolemic view that the earth was at the center of the universe (based on the beliefs of astronomer Ptolemy) to the Copernican view that the sun is the center of the universe (based on the beliefs of astronomer Nicolaus Copernicus) is a classic ex-ample of a paradigm shift—it caused a lot of pain and took centuries to take hold. (Copernicus did not release his theory of a sun-centered universe until he was on his deathbed for fear of persecution!)

> As with any paradigm shift, the magnitude of change is massive, the resistance strong, and the shift itself years in the making.

It won't take centuries or a deathbed revelation (I hope) for hospital marketers to fully embrace this paradigm shift, but it won't take only a few years either. The behaviors that sup-port the existing paradigm have been around for decades, or, essentially, since the beginning of the hospital marketing industry in the 1980s. That won't change overnight. It takes time to overcome the biases, the beliefs, the entrenched in-terests, and the incentives that grew out of the existing paradigm. It's safe to say that jobs, if not entire positions and industry sectors, are at stake here.

Nonetheless, the correct paradigm wins out—it always does. And in fact, we are making progress, and there are hospital and health system marketers who *have* embraced the new paradigm. Not only embraced it but made the shift from old to new, marketers who are *operating* in the new paradigm, not just aspiring to it. They have forged ahead and are—at least in terms of rejecting mass, promotional marketing for digital and content marketing—working in ways that are diametrically opposed to the status quo in our industry.

This book is for those who also want to operate within the new paradigm but aren't exactly sure how to go about it or what the "new world" might look like. If you're unsure of the need to make this transition, go back and read *Joe Public One* or any of the subsequent stories, blog posts, podcasts, or presentations I've put out supporting that transition in the few years since the book was released. But if you're ready to jump off the deep end and really—I mean *really, truly*—embrace change, let this book be your guide. This is an attempt to paint that picture of the other side for you: What will you be doing differently? What changes will you make? What will it look like? What will it feel like? How will you know you're there?

THE STRUCTURE OF THIS BOOK

At this point, the goal is clear: move from a worldview that emphasizes mass, promotional advertising campaigns to one that prioritizes digital marketing and content marketing. But these paradigms are structured differently, and it's important to understand those differences at the outset.

First, we're defining the existing paradigm as the merging of its two components—mass advertising and promotional messaging. You can have mass advertising and you can have promotional messaging, and separately they can be wielded effectively for good. It's when they are combined and given such prominence that they become the most overused, abused, misused, ineffective form of marketing in our industry. This unholy combination is easy to see in our industry, as billboards with five stars and television ads with smiling nurses extend as far as the eye can see. Of course, there is a place for strategically intentioned, effective mass advertising campaigns wielding promotional messages. It's not the practice itself that is bad; it's the way we as an industry rely too much on this terribly expensive, terribly ineffective approach that is the problem. (Later, in Chapter 8, I'll describe a little of why we are so addicted to the old paradigm.) So the old paradigm is something easily identified, and it is easily defined as the linking of two components—mass advertising and promotional messaging.

The new paradigm, however, requires the consideration of its core elements—digital marketing (instead of mass advertising) and content marketing (instead of promotional marketing)—separately. It's not that you wouldn't leverage digital marketing in a content marketing effort—you most certainly would. But to fully master and leverage each component, they should be thought of separately.

Furthermore, the ways in which we should approach these two elements varies dramatically. Digital marketing constitutes a fundamental shift in thinking, approach, goals, tools, channels, budget and resource allocation, staffing skill sets, and measurement. Mastering digital marketing requires at least an understanding of dozens if not hundreds of variant applications, from the ever-expanding list of social media channels to location-based services, to mobile to website design, to CRM and CMS and SEO and SEM. The complexity involved is mind-boggling, the scope as broad as an ocean, the landscape ever-changing.

Content marketing, on the other hand, is a much simpler change to understand and master. As we will see, there is really only one primary philosophy that needs to change, with subsequent changes in operation and execution flowing naturally from there. If digital marketing is 100 miles wide and 100 miles long and 100 miles deep, content marketing is one square mile that goes maybe 10 miles deep. That is not to say, however, that embracing content marketing is easier than embracing digital marketing. The one philosophical change required is so contrarian to our world and to what many in our organization believe is effective that content marketing can in some ways be more difficult to pursue than digital marketing.

Reflecting this reality, I've split the book into two parts: Part One—Digital Marketing Mastery, and Part Two—Content Marketing Mastery. I've approached digital marketing in this book in a leveled, hierarchical way, providing an overview of the digital marketing mindset in Chapter 2 and attributes of digital mastery in Chapter 3. Content marketing, on the other hand, is covered in a more linear fashion in Chapter 6. To seal the deal, each section features a case study demonstrating how a healthcare organization has achieved success in the new consumer healthcare marketing paradigm.

As you'll see, there is much overlap between the two, and they do share one significant trait—they can be extremely difficult to pursue given the obstacles you're likely to encounter within your own organization. That's why we follow Parts One and Two with a chapter on preparing your organization for the new healthcare marketing paradigm.

WHO IS THIS BOOK FOR?

Before we go any further, it's worth identifying exactly whom I had in mind when I wrote this book. For starters, this book is for those who work at provider healthcare organizations—health systems, hospitals, clinics, etc. Many of the principles will apply to other healthcare organizations, but the content found here was developed for those in marketing, communications, strategy, digital/interactive and public relations at provider organizations.

If you are either unaware of the arguments made in *Joe Public One* or are aware of them but don't agree they are necessary, this book is likely not for you. While I spend a little time here and there building the case for the overall concept of embracing the new consumer healthcare marketing paradigm, I'm assuming you are already on board with the idea that moving away from mass, promotional advertising is smart. If you aren't, I'm not sure this book makes sense for you. If you're already operating under the new paradigm—congratulations! You're on your way, and you may not need all of the guidelines provided here, but you may find some new ideas or strategies. Finally, this isn't a book on SEO, content strategy, website design, or any of those specific areas. It's a book on how to appropriately leverage elements of digital marketing and content marketing in a strategic way to drive better marketing and branding results. Even if you're an expert in one area, learning how your area fits with the rest under the new paradigm might still be worth a read. But if you're looking to dive deep into any of these specific areas, this isn't the place.

Which leaves you, fair reader. The person who craves change but isn't sure how to make it happen. The person who explores digital marketing, who leverages social media, who desires a more mobile-savvy approach but isn't sure how to master it. The person who would like to know how to move mass, promotional advertising campaigns to the appropriate position on the list (typically near the end) and instead use robust content-marketing programs to build brand and drive volumes. The person who yearns to cross the bridge from old to new and become an industry leader. This is your time, and this is your book.

ABOUT ANOTHER BIG CHANGE

Some would argue that there's an even more significant shift occurring than the one I reference in this book—a shift that will have an even more dramatic impact on the role of marketers in hospitals and health systems. That's the industry move away from the fee-for-service model to a model borne of the Affordable Care Act (ACA), a model emphasizing fee-for-quality, accountable care, and population health management. I have heard some marketers claim that because of this shift, the purview of healthcare marketers will fundamentally move from one of finding and attracting the right patients to one of keeping patients and populations healthy and well. That rather than pulling patients in, our jobs will be to keep them out.

ACA and the industry changes it is driving appear to be here to stay and will no doubt have a lasting impact on how care is delivered in this country, if the changes I'm seeing at organizations across the country hold up. Maybe I'm being the stubborn old-schooler now, but I personally do not believe this will fundamentally change the role of hospital and healthcare marketers. Will marketers now have to consider health and wellness messaging, population health efforts, and increased/enhanced patient education? Most likely yes, though to split hairs, those responsibilities would be better defined as "communication responsibilities" rather than marketing responsibilities. Will those responsibilities outweigh or even completely replace the traditional marketing responsibilities? I don't think so.

That's because for all of the change the ACA is driving, it doesn't alter the fact that clinics, hospitals, and health systems still need to attract and care for the right patients to stay financially viable. When we say we want to "keep patients out of the hospital," this is true in the sense that we don't want patients returning to the hospital post-treatment for unnecessary readmissions lest we suffer the reimbursement penalties that would draw. And the system would certainly benefit from eliminating misguided and expensive fee-for-service incentives, allowing us to care for people in the most appropriate way possible. But we will still need to care for people. Hospitals still need reimbursable encounters to generate the revenue

> The ACA doesn't change the fact that hospitals need to find and attract the right patients and that consumers have a choice of where to receive care, meaning hospitals still need to compete for those patients.

(if not net profit) needed to keep their doors open. The ACA doesn't change the fact that hospitals need to find and attract the right patients and that consumers have a choice of where to receive care, meaning hospitals still need to compete for those patients. And hospitals will still need a strong and differentiated brand to achieve those goals.

Those are all goals served by marketing, which respected marketing guru Philip Kotler defines as "the art of finding, developing, and profiting from opportunities." Unless our national health system shifts to a public utility model, where the government mandates hospitals to serve a specific geographic population, and *only* that population, with consumers having no choice as to where they receive care (as usually occurs with electricity, gas, and cable services), there will always be a need for hospitals and health systems to employ marketing expertise to find, develop, and profit from care opportunities (with "profit" being a relative word— even nonprofit organizations need to take in more money than they spend).

This book is designed to show hospitals and health systems how to use digital and content-oriented strategies to pursue more effective marketing results. The good news is that what you learn here about digital marketing and content marketing will also be invaluable in helping you, if you're so tasked, with supporting patient education and population health efforts. So you're covered either way.

PART ONE

DIGITAL MARKETING MASTERY

CHAPTER 1

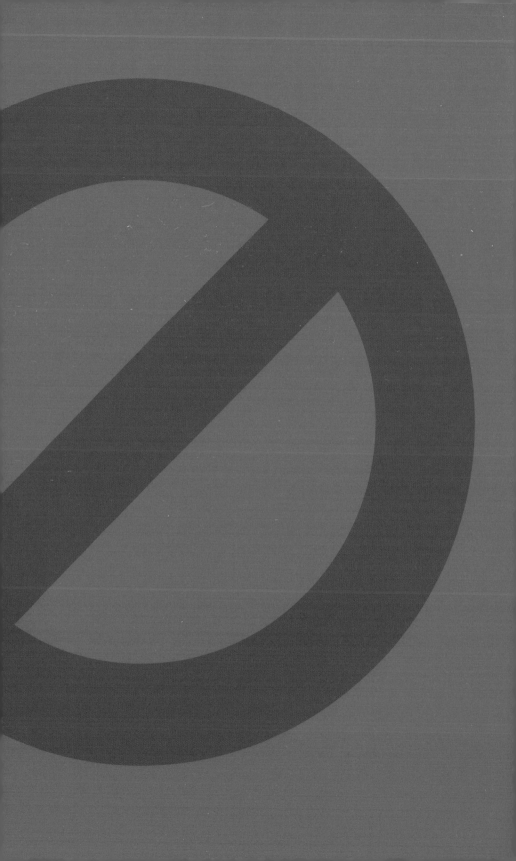

BREAKING OUR ADDICTION TO MASS ADVERTISING

YOU HAD ME AT HELLO

In late 2012, I wrote what I called my "Jerry Maguire" memo to the healthcare marketing industry. The blog post, which was a response to a published industry story on why hospitals needed to advertise themselves and their services on a mass scale, was really a rant against the old paradigm of healthcare marketing. As such, it's worth revisiting because, to embrace the new paradigm, we must shake ourselves free of one of the foundations of the old paradigm—mass marketing. This exorcism then sets the stage for the most critical aspect of the new paradigm: *digital marketing mastery.*

··········

If you don't remember your 1990s movies, *Jerry Maguire* was an Academy Award–nominated movie starring Tom Cruise playing a sports agent going through something of a midlife crisis. At the outset of the film, Cruise's character issues a memo titled "The Things We Think and Do Not Say: The Future of Our Business" at a conference lamenting the way the industry has evolved and wishing for a return to more personalized relationships with clients. Realizing the errors of the industry's ways, he calls out his fellow agents, turning reformer and casting a critical light on the very business that made him a success. My advocacy for the new consumer healthcare marketing paradigm is my Jerry Maguire memo to the healthcare marketing industry.

I've had my marketing firm for nearly 20 years, and for the majority of that time we've worked only with healthcare organizations, and primarily hospitals and health systems. Up until just a couple of years ago, I can tell you that my firm generated more revenue from creating hospital mass advertising than from any other source. Yet since the release of *Joe Public One* in 2011, I've been traveling the country, speaking at conferences, pleading with clients, telling anyone who will listen—for the love of all that's holy, put mass advertising at the back of the line.

Right now, of course, mass advertising is often the first tactic out of the gate for hospital marketers. The latest By the Numbers survey from SHSMD shows that, once again, hospitals spend more money on mass advertising than on any other marketing expense. But you don't need a survey to tell you that. Just drive around any of our cities and behold the hospital billboards, one after another after another. View the ubiquitous television, listen to the plethora of radio spots, and gaze upon the sea of print ads. Doesn't it blow your mind that, as an industry, our number-one choice of marketing tactic—mass advertising—is the same as the number-one choice in 1974? Literally four decades have passed, and while other industries are adapting to new marketing strategies, channels, and tools, we're stuck in the past.

Now, I'm the first to stand up and defend a hospital's right to market itself, and that includes mass advertising. We have a market-driven system, and I believe that competition and choice can deliver a better healthcare system than a socialized, government-run version. But that's a moot argument for now—as long as we have a market-driven system, hospitals and other providers must be allowed to compete for patients. But just because we can use mass advertising as a means to compete doesn't mean we *should* use it in such overwhelmingly ineffective ways.

The arguments in defense of hospital mass advertising have been around for as long as I've been in this business. In fact, I have used many of them myself to defend the practice in the past. But our world has changed. Our country can no longer sustain the ways we currently deliver healthcare, so reform is upon us. Accountable care, shrinking reimbursements, public health responsibilities, organizational efficiencies. From a marketing perspective, new tools such as the Internet, social media, and mobile technology have emerged, and we have more sophisticated strategies and systems to help us understand how to drive much more effective marketing results. We have to think differently.

Let's take these oft-repeated arguments in support of hospital mass advertising one by one and finally, once and for all, push aside the past and move toward a more effective future.

1. Mass advertising as patient education

There are two sides to this. Patient education regarding public health issues, wellness, and other health-oriented content is a good thing. But the vast majority of hospitals use patient education from an advertising perspective to "educate" consumers about the services they offer and/or why those services are different or better than other choices in the market. In other words, education equals self-promotion. Marketers often lament that without mass advertising, how would community members know what services are available to them?

This would be the equivalent of Walmart claiming that its advertising is essential to educating consumers about the product choices available to them in the market. Let's be real—this isn't about education; it's about selling. Walmart knows it, consumers know it, hospital marketers know it—we all know it.

I agree that consumers do need to understand the healthcare choices that are available to them. That's essential to a market-driven, competitive ecosystem. But do we have to spend millions in paid mass advertising to do it? Let's dream for a minute. Wouldn't it be great if we had a centralized resource that consumers could turn to when they need care? A place they could look for all the options in their market, compare their choices, conduct research, and talk to others about their opinions of the market options? A place that was free and easily accessible, such as through a home-based appliance—the stove, or maybe a blender. Oh wait, we do have something like that—the Internet, available through your computer, tablet, or phone (and coming soon, your blender). That's what consumers are using to learn about their choices and become "educated." We've all seen the studies showing that the majority of people go online for information about their health. We don't need to spend millions on billboards and TV spots to educate consumers. It's not 1974 anymore.

2. The business case

Here's my favorite claim about the value of hospital advertising: "Hospitals need to advertise to maintain or enhance revenue flow." This is similar to a quote I recently heard from a CEO (which, I'd guess, has been repeated time and again in hospitals across the country): "Where is our advertising? We need to get out there and generate business!" Really? Advertising is how we generate business? That's how we drive new patients in? It's not the experience we deliver or the access we provide to an important service in a neighborhood that needs it? Or building strong physician referral channels or well-placed urgent care and emergency centers? Or showing up in search results when a consumer jumps online? Or having a website that is clear, easy to navigate, and provides the information they need? Or offering health and wellness content that draws consumers in based on what's relevant to them and their situation? No, of course not. Running a radio spot promoting your board-certified general surgeon is the surest way to drive general surgery volumes.

Of course advertising can drive some patients in. But in healthcare, people don't think about us until they need us. We are not a demand-driven industry. I don't care how fantastic your billboard is, it can't make someone have gall bladder removal surgery. The truth is, the vast majority of people in any market are not shopping for what you're selling because they don't need care. Put another way, *Joe Public Doesn't Care About Your Hospital.* So, sure, you can run a TV campaign talking about your da Vinci robot and get the attention of the seven people who at that moment are considering where to receive robotic surgery. But your message is wasted on the other 100,000 people who don't need surgery and thus don't care about your robot. Aren't there more effective and less costly ways to find those seven people? And while we're at it, aren't there more effective ways to actually impact the other 100,000? It's not about you or your services; it's about them— what is relevant to those in your market who don't need care today but inevitably will tomorrow.

In fact, the business case for hospital advertising—especially mass advertising—is extraordinarily poor. It's notoriously difficult to measure the impact of the ubiquitous "brand campaigns" that are all about awareness and perception building and have no call to action. But the effectiveness of mass advertising from a cost/benefit perspective pales in comparison to more targeted efforts, such as search advertising, direct mail, or community seminars. Yes, some of that is advertising, but it's the mass advertising that's getting us in trouble. Billboards, radio, TV—you hear me? We're coming for you.

3. But advertising is just a tiny portion of the operating budget

Very true. Even for big-spending systems, a large, multi-channel mass advertising campaign is what I like to call a pimple on the butt of the overall operating budget. But does that excuse the practice, especially when we realize how gosh-darn ineffective it is? Spending a million dollars to promote the message of "We care," or letting folks know that your team of arm-crossing orthopods "has your back" is still a waste of money regardless of how tiny a piece of the pie it is. From a marketing perspective, imagine what you could do with the million dollars that was wasted on flashy, chest-pounding ads. Create a fantastic interactive experience? Offer community education on diabetes, weight loss, or stress reduction? Buy cloth robes for breast cancer patients? Develop compelling, relevant health and wellness content? Offer a dozen online health risk assessments? The list of ways to truly engage your audiences—not just yap at them—goes on and on.

Of course there are circumstances when mass advertising makes sense. Building awareness for a new clinic, for example, or launching a new brand in a market. But I think it's fair to say that the vast majority of hospital ads are doing little or nothing to support the organizations that run them. In this day and age, with our bloated national healthcare system wasting billions of dollars on an annual basis, any significant inefficiency should be reconsidered. Self-promoting mass advertising is an easy choice because it is wasteful. If you don't want to be in a negative media spotlight, stop wasting money that could be better spent.

The truth is, the above oft-cited "logical" reasons supporting mass advertising are only partly responsible for its abuse and overuse. For many marketers, it's what they know, it's what they've always done, it's relatively easy, it can be fun, and it's the biggest way to raise their own personal profile. ("Look at this awesome TV spot we created!") We have seen the enemy, and she is us. Many ad agencies still have business models built on mass advertising and the media commissions they drive, so they are constantly pounding the marketing nail with a mass advertising hammer. But perhaps the biggest driver of mass advertising is the pressure applied by physicians, administrators, and others who don't understand marketing and believe filling their beds is as simple as erecting a billboard. "We're a hidden gem! Go tell our story! We need business! Where's our billboard?" More marketing dollars have been burned trying to assuage the politically powerful and those with little or no marketing education or expertise in our organizations than I care to count. These are the true reasons mass advertising is still the number-one marketing tactic for hospitals. And none of them hold up to the scrutiny of doing what's right, both for marketing effectiveness and for the communities we serve.

So let's pursue what *is* right. Let's master digital marketing.

CHAPTER 2

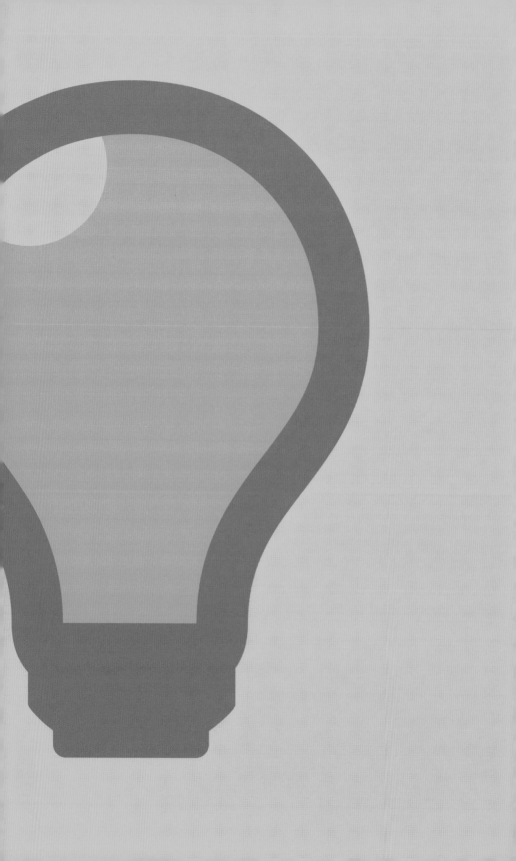

THE DIGITAL MARKETING MIND-SET

THE SNAKE THAT EATS ITS TAIL

OK, that's off my chest. I feel better. Do you? Hopefully that rousing rant will allow you to move into what is perhaps the most challenging aspect of embracing the new healthcare marketing paradigm—mastering digital marketing. To accomplish that, you have to understand and embrace the digital marketing *mind-set*. What's interesting about this mind-set is that once you achieve it, you will no longer have a need for it. (Say what?)

There's a reason I still call my firm, Interval, a healthcare *marketing* firm rather than a healthcare *digital marketing* firm, even though the vast majority of work we do for clients is digital in nature. Our focus, like yours, is to employ successful marketing strategies for hospitals and health systems. There are many types of marketing strategies, and many more components to support those strategies. Today, it just so happens that the more effective strategies and components are digital in nature. That doesn't mean, however, that you abandon the nondigital strategies and components—events, direct marketing, heck, even mass advertising still can serve a purpose. Digital is a means to an end—marketing success—not the end in and of itself.

Yet our industry is still in a place where digital is carved out and thought of in a distinct way. To demonstrate this point, let's use a nonsensical example with something we're all familiar with—billboards. Let's imagine that up until 2010, outdoor advertising didn't exist. No billboards, no bus sides, no posters, no nothing. Then imagine that in 2010, some genius dreams up the idea of advertising messages delivered on outdoor platforms, and suddenly, outdoor advertising is an option for hospital marketers. At first, there would be a rush to understand this new medium: How can it be leveraged? What are best practices for using outdoor advertising venues? How do the benefits of a billboard match those of a bus-stop poster? Consultants would emerge with specific outdoor expertise, and marketing departments would begin hiring specialists to focus on outdoor marketing. Books would be written on how to master outdoor marketing. Hospital CMOs would develop "outdoor strategies" to answer board members and C-suiters demanding to know "what are we doing about outdoor?!?" Some hospitals would rush headlong into embracing outdoor advertising, maybe creating positions such as "vice president of outdoor," while others would move cautiously, unconvinced of the new medium's worth.

All of this should sound familiar—in many ways, it reflects our industry's current approach to digital marketing. It's a fairly nascent discipline that we're all struggling to understand and use effectively. And the questions and behaviors in the fake scenario described above are understandable, given the emergence of a new field. But now play this fake scenario out. Once the industry learned the value of outdoor advertising, its role in the overall marketing mix, and the pros and cons of various types of outdoor advertising, would it then make sense to think of outdoor advertising distinctly from other marketing media? Would you need a "vice president of outdoor" or a distinct outdoor advertising strategy? Given what we know about outdoor advertising in the real world, that sounds kind of silly. And yet isn't that where we could end up eventually with digital?

Let's look at one way this dynamic plays out with digital today. We've been approached by many organizations to develop a digital strategy—it's actually one of our firm's primary offerings. What do clients mean by a digital strategy? In the vast majority of cases, hospitals and health systems are already doing some kind of digital marketing. Many have been using social media for a few years or have been incorporating direct email communications as a part of a service line program. Perhaps the organization's website has received a much-needed face-lift, or maybe pay-per-click advertising has been employed.

But what often leads to the call for a digital strategy is marketing leaders' recognition that these tools and tactics don't live in isolation and that an overarching approach is needed to maximize the benefit of all digital marketing efforts. In looking at a digital strategy, organizations typically include everything from website functionality to mobile to video production—anything that can be used or shared in a digital channel or format. But here's the issue: Just as it would be wrong to build a marketing strategy that includes only outdoor tactics, it is also misguided to develop a strategy that includes *only* digital tactics. It is an oxymoronic, snake-eating-its-tail, mind-bending point—**to master digital marketing, you want to get to a place where you no longer think about digital in terms of a distinct strategy, tool, or channel.** Those strategies, tools, and channels that are digital in nature will just become components of the overall marketing mix and won't be carved out because of their digital nature. Thus, the ultimate goal of your digital journey is to kill, once and for all, the need to think about digital separately at all. This doesn't mean you won't have people on your team who are focused on digital—a website manager, SEO consultant, or social media specialist. What it means is that as the marketing leader, you will no longer create separate "digital strategies," have distinct "digital plans," or think in terms of "how can we use digital to support this effort?"

> To master digital marketing, you want to get to a place where you no longer think about digital in terms of a distinct strategy, tool, or channel.

That's your final destination—that's real digital marketing mastery. But you're not there yet, and until you are, you **do** have to think about and understand digital as a distinct entity. If digital marketing mastery is your end goal, then adopting a digital marketing mind-set is how you get there. Truth is, it will be years before you can achieve digital marketing mastery, and the marketing industry itself will take even longer to evolve to the point that digital is just woven into the fabric of marketing rather than being treated as a distinct entity.

So you have to develop a digital marketing mind-set to best leverage the various digital strategies, tools, and channels at your disposal. How do you develop such a mind-set?

HOW THE DIGITAL MARKETING MIND-SET IS LIKE HAVING KIDS

For starters, a little perspective may help. If you're like most healthcare marketers, you're employing some type of digital marketing—you have a Facebook page, you buy pay-per-click advertising, you have videos on your website, and so on. So you may be thinking that developing a digital marketing mind-set is about *increasing* your digital marketing efforts. You realize you need to do more with digital, and you're thinking, "How will embracing the digital marketing mind-set *add* to what I'm already doing in terms of budget, resources, or time spent?" But the digital marketing mind-set goes well beyond incremental—or even substantial—increases in time, money, or effort. It will completely change your approach to marketing.

Those of you with kids will understand this difference if you think back to before you had kids and to how you likely imagined what life would be like with children. How much more time would you need to devote to your family? Would that limit your free time or the time you could spend on your career? How much more money would it cost? How would that impact the other priorities in your life in terms of money, such as the house you want to buy or saving for retirement? You questioned friends and family, wanting to know how your life would change. And you likely received a smile and a shake of the head: "There's no way to describe how your life changes until it happens to you." That's because when you have kids, you certainly *do* experience significant changes in the time and money you spend. But more dramatically, having kids completely changes your worldview, far beyond easily measured components such as time and money. How you think about the world changes, what matters to you changes, your approach to life changes. And it's not an exaggeration to say that once you cross the great divide to digital marketing mastery, the same fundamental level of change will occur in you. Your entire approach to marketing will never be the same.

SIX KEYS TO THE DIGITAL MARKETING MIND-SET

How do you achieve the digital marketing mind-set? Certainly, embracing digital involves understanding and leveraging the myriad tools and channels that digital offers. You'll learn more about these in Chapter 4. But learning to be a master of SEO or social media is not enough. Since I'm such a huge fan of analogies, here's another to help make this point.

Let's say you're building a new home, and you know you will need someone to handle drywalling. You can find someone who has spent years learning to drywall, who has become the best in the land at "drywall mastery." You hire this master to work on your new home. But without a strong design, clear architectural blueprint, and smart general contracting management to oversee the building of your new home, that expert can put all of his years of experience to work only to find out that he's been drywalling in the wrong place.

By the same token, you can become an expert in SEO, social media, or whatever, but without understanding how to leverage those tools in the great scheme of digital marketing, and even more important, in *marketing overall*, you will never maximize the use of those tools.

Here are six key principles, in no intentional order, to help you achieve the digital marketing mind-set. These are by no means the only components of a digital marketing mind-set, but they are the steps most important in helping to shift from the old paradigm to the new. In the next chapter, you will learn more about the channels, tools, and resources you need to understand. Finally, in Chapter 4, I'll help show you what it looks and feels like once you've arrived.

1 **Change your frame of reference regarding digital marketing tools and channels, moving from thinking about them secondarily and separately to considering them initially and integrated.**

Because many of the digital channels and tools available to us are so new, they are often an afterthought from a marketing perspective. How often does this happen in your marketing department...

You've been tasked with a strategic marketing goal—raising cardiology volumes. Your team assembles and follows a marketing planning process, learning more about the specific needs of the cardiology department, such as desired goals and objectives, key audiences, types of services to feature, and more. You build a plan to market cardiology, including a multi-channel consumer campaign focused on your new heart center, featuring a series of educational seminars on heart health held throughout the community. The creative team is engaged, a campaign is developed, and at some point, someone realizes your campaign will need a website landing page. So you approach your digital team with direction on what's needed for the landing page and give them a two-week deadline to create and launch the page.

That, my friends, is old-school thinking. As we'll discuss in a bit, your website should be the center of all your marketing efforts. As such, those responsible for it should play a role upfront in the planning and creative phase rather than being handed an assignment in the execution phase. As you adopt the digital marketing mind-set, the use of digital marketing channels and tools will become a driving force for your planning and creative efforts rather than an afterthought.

2   **Move away from developing plans or strategies that are "digital" focused. Instead, integrate digital channels and resources throughout your marketing planning efforts.**

We've already discussed how a smart digital strategy, by its nature, has a self-destruct mechanism built in: At the point you achieve digital marketing mastery, you will no longer think of "digital marketing" separately but will simply see it as "marketing."

For example, instead of having a traditional media plan (which is focused primarily on traditional media outlets) separate from a search engine marketing (SEM) plan or other digital advertising plan, consider creating an integrated media plan that encompasses all paid media.

In typical healthcare organizations, everyone in a marketing and communications function touches digital in some way, and there may be few roles dedicated solely or primarily to digital content, tools, or resources. As you grow into a digital marketing mind-set, it may be helpful to designate someone to wear the "digital" hat during marketing planning processes for at least a certain amount of time to ensure that digital marketing options are constantly and effectively considered. Eventually, everyone in the department will have a "digitally driven" perspective, and the ultimate goal – digital marketing becoming thought of simply as "marketing" – will be achieved.

3 **When developing specific marketing plans or campaigns, start with three areas—web, mobile, and search—before considering any other tactic (digital or otherwise).**

We tell our clients that with any significant marketing initiative—a service-line marketing program, a brand-building campaign, a new specialty clinic launch—the first three priorities should be interactive, search, and mobile. Why is that? Because the biggest challenge we have in healthcare marketing is being front and center with consumers when they need our services. If you are looking for a new physician, are exploring different cancer treatment options, or need knee surgery, where's the first place you turn? Research shows that people turn to their spouses, parents, friends, coworkers, and, today, our trusted social media networks. Word of mouth is the most powerful of drivers for healthcare decision making, which is why your brand experience and social media strategies are so crucial. What's next? The vast majority of those seeking information on healthcare choices turn to Google (or Yelp, or Facebook, or Siri...). So when a consumer is ready to look for you, you'd better be there, ranked high on organic search engine result pages (SERPs) and in targeted search engine advertising.

And when they search for and find you, where's the first place they go? Your website. That means you need a compelling and intuitive interactive experience that provides relevant content, engaging tools, and a clear path to action. We've heard it a million times—your website is your new front door. Yet how many hospitals and health systems still have a hot mess for a website? An increasing number of consumers are now searching for and experiencing your website from their phone or tablet. According to many experts, within the next couple of years, more people will access the Internet from a mobile device than from a desktop computer. But you're ready for that, with a responsive website, accurate location listings, and location-based activity, right? Moving forward, challenge yourself to explore these and other more effective marketing avenues (such as customer relationship management programs, direct marketing and events) before falling back to the standby of mass advertising.

4 Learn how to incorporate digital marketing channels, resources, and efforts effectively from both a horizontal and vertical standpoint.

As followers of my articles, books, and podcast undoubtedly know, the team at Interval likes to make up new terms, concepts and definitions to help illustrate a point or phenomenon ("left side of the menu" marketing, anyone?) One of the dynamics we've seen with those wanting to embrace the new consumer healthcare marketing paradigm is how they struggle to wrap their arms around digital marketing. So many channels, so many strategies, so many tools—how do you put them all in perspective? How do you prioritize your efforts? How do you avoid pursuing digital "for digital's sake?"

Horizontal and vertical perspectives

To help marketers grapple with those questions, we've created another new concept—applying horizontal and vertical perspectives to your digital marketing efforts. Knowing the difference between these perspectives will help you better understand how to maximize digital channels, tools, and resources.

We define horizontal as ongoing efforts that exist regardless of current marketing goals, strategies, or objectives. For example, regardless of your current marketing goals, your organization must have an effective website and a strong social media presence. The same isn't true of some traditional marketing resources such as outdoor advertising or community events. Vertical is defined as serving a specific marketing goal or effort. So while you need a strong, ongoing social media presence, the ways in which you leverage social media from this horizontal perspective may vary from the ways you leverage social media to support a vertical initiative, such as targeting women age 35+ or creating a campaign to build cardiac volumes in your market.

> So many channels, so many strategies, so many tools—how do you put them all in perspective?

On the following page you will find an example of horizontal/vertical thinking applied to Search Engine Marketing (SEM)...

VERTICAL

Advanced

PPC on Bing, Yahoo, other search engines

Event-based PPC

Testing

Creative-based A/B testing

Location-based A/B testing

Basics

Heart disease HRA PPC

Heart health/education PPC

Procedure-specific PPC

Extended CV physician PPC

HORIZONTAL

Competitive blocking

Physician-based PPC

Location-based PPC

Search Engine Marketing

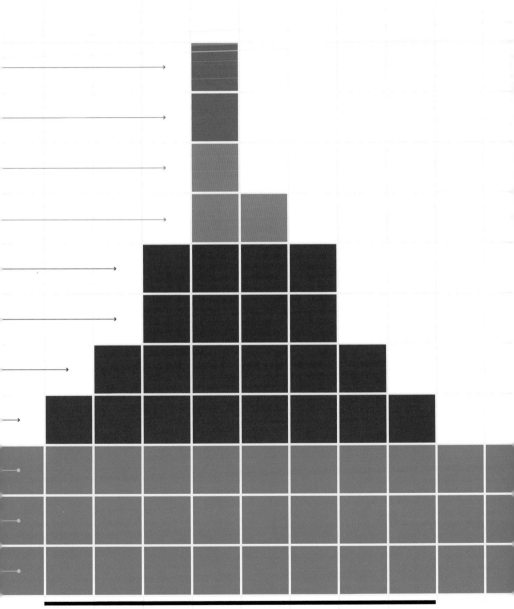

Cardiology marketing program

Sophisticated hospital marketers have an ongoing SEM strategy to ensure that those searching for location- or time-sensitive services, such urgent care clinics or emergency rooms, will always be able to find our locations through effective pay-per-click. In some cases, hospitals will run competitive SEM efforts to ensure that users see their ads when searching specifically for a competing facility. This is an example of appropriate horizontal marketing using SEM—it happens on a continuous basis, regardless of your top marketing priorities. After all, SEM is the low-hanging fruit of healthcare marketing—it allows you to place yourself directly in front of someone who is seeking medical advice, information, or services. That's pretty much the holy grail of healthcare marketing, and hospitals should always seek to leverage this strategy.

Now imagine that your organization's marketing plan calls for a campaign targeting women age 35+. Your SEM campaigns could be developed to focus on certain health issues (high-risk pregnancies or menopause, for example) or clinical needs (breast cancer or incontinence, for example). These would be appropriate vertical marketing efforts using SEM, enacted to support a strategic marketing effort.

Avoiding digital "for the sake of digital"

Thinking about digital marketing in terms of horizontal and vertical applications will help you better prioritize your efforts. For example, while you always want to have some sort of SEM effort running, you may save your more significant investments in SEM for your highest-priority marketing efforts. In addition, understanding how and when to apply horizontal and vertical thinking will help you avoid the trap of using digital "for the sake of digital." Let's look at SEM again as an example of this misguided approach.

Some organizations might try to use SEM to target situations in which people are searching for help in areas that may be difficult to promote using traditional channels, such as the treatment of sexually transmitted diseases. This is an example of thinking about the channel or tool first, rather than leveraging the channel or tool for a strategic purpose. Unless the SEM campaign supports a horizontal marketing need (location-based targeting or competitive blocking, for example) or a vertical marketing need (the goal to reach women age 35+ or to support a large cardiovascular marketing campaign), the digital effort probably isn't strategic in nature and thus should be avoided.

Other examples of using digital "for the sake of digital" that we've seen include the following:

- Pursuing additional video production because "we need more videos on the website"
- Creating a mobile app because it's cool to have a mobile app
- Jumping on the hot new social media channel without a well-thought-out strategy or the ability to commit to a certain level of engagement

Trying to leverage digital "for the sake of digital" is the equivalent of trying to leverage billboards "for the sake of outdoor." Imagine asking, "There are 20 billboards in our community—how should we use them?" rather than letting your marketing plan, strategies, or priorities drive whether billboards are appropriate.

Getting a grip

If you're struggling to get a grip on how to leverage digital marketing, using horizontal and vertical perspectives is a simple framework you can use to guide your team's activities, build strategies, and set marketing priorities. Not only will it help you avoid applying digital "for the sake of digital," but it's a critical component of a digital mind-set that maximizes the effectiveness of your overall marketing and helps to ensure that you're supporting your organization's goals in the best way possible.

5 In all marketing (but particularly digital marketing) seek to always drive engagement as the ultimate goal.

To maximize the effects of digital marketing channels, resources, and efforts, marketers must move beyond the goals of building awareness and perception.

One of the great afflictions of our industry when it comes to marketing is what I call the hidden gem syndrome. This is the belief that we are "unique/different/better/awesome/the best" and that if people just knew that, we'd have all the patients we can handle. The hidden gem syndrome most often affects those who don't truly understand healthcare marketing (such as those in the C-suite or physicians), and who believe marketing's top goal should be to build awareness of the organization. So off we go to create a giant campaign to "get our name out" or "tell our story." There are circumstances in which this one-way communication is appropriate, such as when announcing a new organization name following a merger. However, it's safe to say that any marketing that doesn't try to create two-way interaction is missing a tremendous opportunity.

Investing in brand advertising can work in other industries, such as consumer goods. Pepsi spends millions of dollars annually solely on brand advertising, but for good reason. If you're already a Pepsi drinker, exposure to those ads should make you want to go grab a Pepsi out of the fridge or buy a bottle at a convenience store. If you're not a Pepsi drinker, perhaps the constant exposure to its advertising will entice you to try it. But there are two key differences between Pepsi and your healthcare organization. First, Pepsi has hundreds of millions of dollars in its marketing budget, and you do not. Every precious dollar you have needs to be spent as effectively as possible, and while pouring money into brand advertising can have an impact, good results often require years of ongoing exposure, and that impact fades quickly once the effort ends.

Second, as we know, people don't use healthcare services on a daily, weekly, monthly, or even (sometimes) annual basis. The vast majority of clinical offerings do not lend themselves to demand-based marketing. As I said in the last chapter, no billboard, no matter how effective, will lead someone to say, "That looks great—I think I'll have my gall bladder out today."

The key, then, is to move beyond simply driving awareness of your services to engaging consumers in a compelling and relevant way. Engagement simply means having your target audience take action based on your marketing efforts. Instead of simply hoping to change their opinion in some way (greater awareness, brand perception, etc.), you want to change their behavior. Driving engagement enables you to connect with consumers today and maintain that connection until they need care tomorrow. By using strategies such as content marketing and tools such as social media, seminars, and online health assessments, you will capture consumer information that allows you to stay engaged and build on that connection. That, in turn, provides you with measurable results essential to demonstrating the success of your efforts.

These points are especially important in relation to digital marketing. An intrinsic asset of digital channels, tools, and content is that they offer the opportunity to create two-way interactions, initiated through relevant calls to action wherever appropriate. The benefits of engagement are many: Interaction creates a stronger brand connection, can lead to "actionable conversions" (see below for a definition), and helps connect marketing results to financial results (leveraging CRM systems and other methods). Organizations that leverage digital marketing efforts solely to build awareness (e.g., using online display advertising to "build brand") are missing the true value of digital marketing offers. That doesn't mean you won't impact awareness or perception with digital marketing efforts. But the end goal of digital marketing efforts should never be awareness or perception building alone.

Here are some steps you can take to make engagement a priority in your marketing efforts:

- Start every marketing effort with the following question: What do we want our target audiences to *do*? Contrast that with striving to influence what audiences *think*, which is typically measured by improvements in awareness or perception. The answers may vary, and there may be multiple calls to action, but those actions should be the foundation for measuring success.

- Whenever possible, develop marketing efforts to drive "actionable conversions." By conversion, we mean you've turned unknown visitors to your website or unnamed attendees at your joint pain seminar into known individuals. Because they've taken a specific action, such as requesting information, registering for a webinar, or taking an online risk assessment, you know their name, contact information, and possibly more. By actionable, we mean you've collected this information in a way that, with the individuals' permission, you can take action with them specifically. Maybe you can follow up on a poor risk-assessment score with a phone call. Maybe you can send them an e-newsletter. Maybe you can invite them to other community seminars. The actionable conversion is needed to continue marketing to the individuals in relevant ways.

- Consider that different audiences may need different engagement opportunities, even within the same focused marketing effort. For example, one woman attracted by a breast health campaign may seek an online health risk assessment to determine her potential risk for breast cancer, while another might be interested in a community seminar on the subject, while yet another may be ready to schedule a mammogram. Your marketing efforts should strive to emphasize calls to action that focus on relevant engagement opportunities based on specific content and context.

- Stop quoting impressions of any kind as a metric of marketing success. Impressions are a factor of your effort, not a result or outcome. Would you ever claim a campaign is successful because you distributed 10,000 brochures? Unlikely, though that's the same principle at play when pointing to "one million online impressions." Here's how I approached this misguided thinking in my 2009 book, *A Marketer's Guide to Measuring Results*[1]:

  > In truth, advertising impressions are a function of the media buy and do not necessarily correlate with desired outcomes. For starters, defining 'impression' can be very tricky. Is the impression of someone driving 70

mph on the interstate passing a billboard set among many other billboards the same as the impression of a Web surfer who visits a site when a banner ad rotates through? Perhaps more importantly, an impression does not automatically trigger a change in awareness, perception or behavior.

6 Apply the right thinking to mobile audiences.

In Chapter 3, I will use the term "mobile-first" to help define what it means to be a digitally driven healthcare marketer. But even the way we think about mobile needs to evolve, at least based on what we see and hear throughout the industry.

The term mobile explicitly implies that we as humans are, well—mobile. Moving, on-the-go, running errands, driving around, not at home or in the office. But if we define mobile this way, based on where the user is, we are limiting our scope of thinking from a marketing perspective, which could cause us to miss the mobile boat altogether.

Imagine Jim, a 45-year-old man who has a family history of heart disease. While watching TV from the comfort of his couch, Jim sees something that triggers him to think about his own heart health. His iPhone is sitting beside him, and he decides to do a quick Google search for heart health. Your organization's website offers a heart assessment, and it pops up in his Google results. Because your organization is located within a few miles of Jim's house, he's familiar with you, so he clicks the link, only to find that the site is not mobile-optimized—or worse yet, done in Flash or another format not supported by mobile devices. He zooms in, zooms out, moves the page over, oops, too far, oh shoot, where did that go? Forget this.

Within only a matter of seconds, you've lost a potential pa-tient because of poor user experience. Maybe Jim would move to his computer, but maybe not. Maybe he'd go back to his search results, stumble through a few more awkward websites, and finally find one that allows a quick, easy-to-use mobile experience. Or even worse, maybe he'll just stop considering his heart health and put it off for a later date. In this scenario, according to <u>research done by Google in 2012</u>,[2] of 1,100 adult smartphone users, 61% of respondents said, "If I don't see what I'm looking for right away on a mo-bile site, I'll quickly move on to another site." And even more, 67% of respondents, said, "A mobile-friendly site makes me more likely to buy a product."

In our scenario, Jim is using a "mobile" device but from the comfort of his couch. He is literally the opposite of mobile. And that's where thinking of mobile as "on-the-go" is dan-gerous. According to <u>additional research by Google</u>,[3] the majority of people using a mobile device do so from their home or office. Some hospitals are completely missing from the mobile experience, while many others offer some sort of slimmed-down mobile website or app that was designed with the stereotypical mobile user in mind—someone on the go, out and about. Their mobile app offers very limited con-tent—directions, maps, hours, a physician directory, and so on. But if your entire web experience is not optimized for mobile with all of the content and tools you offer, you're go-ing to miss folks like Jim who are looking for content beyond the basics.

As marketers, we need to be thinking about how everything that is placed on our website will work on mobile devices. How are you going to make it compatible for the various screen sizes and resolutions of phones, tablets, and everything in between (and beyond)? Healthcare websites must be designed to accommodate the consumer using a mobile device to search for maternity classes or for more information about a hospital's orthopedic offerings. If your site isn't optimized for mobile devices, chances are the consumer will end up looking elsewhere.

To ensure that you're delivering an optimized mobile experience, we recommend using responsive design to build your websites. Responsive design is a specific approach that allows you to develop a website that will visually reformat itself on the fly to accommodate any screen size, creating an experience optimized to the device. So no matter how a user is viewing your site, he or she will have access to all of the content your site offers, organized in a way that maximizes the user. A responsive-designed website would have kept Jim engaged and would likely have resulted in a new patient for your organization.

> If your site isn't optimized for mobile devices, chances are the consumer will end up looking elsewhere.

THE DIGITAL MIND-SET IS ALWAYS EVOLVING

The digital mind-set is a frame of reference, a perspective that allows you to understand not only how to leverage the digital tools, channels, and resources of today but also how to accommodate whatever new comes down the pike. The six principles I've outlined here are just one set of philosophies (there are certainly others that could be added), and over time, the digital marketing landscape will likely evolve to a place where some, if not all, of the principles will become marginalized or fade away altogether as effective guidelines. Take, as one example, the growing influence of marketing automation.

When I speak to non-marketing healthcare executives about the new consumer healthcare marketing paradigm, I'm fascinated by the typical reaction. Most provide a nonchalant "yeah, yeah, that all makes sense," followed by "but what's the next big thing?"

On the one hand, I want to grab them by the lapels and shake them vigorously: "We're still stuck in the old paradigm, struggling to appropriately adopt these new strategies and tools in an effective way, and you want to know what's next?" But on the other hand, at least they are trying to be forward-thinking. So rather than push back, I give them what I believe is the appropriate answer to what will be the next big thing in healthcare marketing: marketing automation.

As those familiar with marketing automation like to say, the approach and supporting technology have been around for years, which is technically true. But as with many other marketing and branding strategies and tools, healthcare has been slow to adopt. And with the rapid growth of marketing automation technology providers such as HubSpot, Marketo, and Eloqua—driven largely by the increasing adoption of content marketing strategies—marketing automation stands poised to become a significant part of the healthcare marketer's arsenal.

Marketing automation can be defined as a set of communication strategies enabled by technology that allows you to connect with individuals in a personalized way based on predetermined behaviors. This is different from customer relationship management (CRM) and CRM-based technology, which, among other things, allow you to manage a database of individuals and target them based on age, gender, income, geography, disease propensity, and other demographics. Instead, marketing automation, working in conjunction with CRM, will allow you to identify how individuals are interacting with your organization and, based on that, communicate with them appropriately and automatically.

Here's an example to illustrate the distinction between marketing automation and CRM, which also demonstrates the power of marketing automation.

One way that hospitals use CRM is to support service line marketing initiatives. Let's say you have a marketing goal of increasing orthopedic surgery volumes, and along with other marketing efforts, you leverage your CRM to generate a list of people in your market who are more likely to suffer from joint pain, such as men and women age 55–65. Using this list, you send an email to the target audience offering three tips for how to ease joint pain, encouraging recipients to go to your website where they can take a free online joint pain risk assessment. While most online risk assessment tools will allow you to send a follow-up email to those who provide their information and complete the assessment, any further connection to those potential patients, let alone those on the original list, must be driven by communications that are manually created and delivered by someone on your marketing team.

Imagine the same scenario, but you've also employed marketing automation as part of your campaign. A short list of the communications you could send might include the following:

- An email to those who didn't take action on your initial email blast, offering additional tips and a second prompt to use the online risk assessment

- An email to those who visited the landing page for the assessment but didn't start it, with a second prompt to do so

- An email to those who started the assessment but didn't finish it, asking if they encountered trouble and encouraging them to complete the task

- An email to those who did complete the assessment and scored low on a potential joint issue risk, inviting them to subscribe to a quarterly email with additional advice on staying healthy

- An email to those who completed the assessment with a high potential for joint issues, encouraging them to talk to their physician or seek out one of yours if they don't have one

- An email to those who scheduled an appointment with one of your physicians, providing directions, parking guidelines, and other appointment-related instructions

- A follow-up email to those who didn't schedule an appointment, encouraging them once again to speak to a physician

In each case, the communication contains content customized to the specific situation described, and the emails are automatically generated based on the triggers and scripts that you developed ahead of time. While emails are used as examples here, marketing automation can trigger any other type of marketing communication as well, such as direct mail or phone calls. Marketing automation even allows you to track the behavior of visitors to your website, tying web activity to individuals with known profiles within your CRM. Once users engage by providing their information using an online form, you can track their behavior using "cookies" assigned by marketing automation technology. In the scenario described above, once a person completes the online risk assessment and provides his or her contact information, you're able to connect the individual's future behavior to his or her personal record. Let's say that person takes no further action in terms of scheduling an appointment or connecting in other ways but continues to return to your orthopedic section over the next few days. Marketing automation allows you to monitor and act on this behavior. You could, for example, configure your content management system and site templates to deliver custom content to that person at the next visit, such as placing a link to a paper on joint pain prominently in a sidebar throughout your orthopedic section, making it easier for that individual to find the information he or she is searching for.

From even this basic example, one can envision the potential implications of marketing automation on healthcare marketing, and on the delivery of healthcare as a whole. Marketing automation allows organizations to fulfill the promise of truly personalized communications, which helps optimize how you move consumers through the funnel from consumer to potential patient to patient. Most marketers spend all of their time, energy, and money trying to connect with audiences in ways they hope will lead to clinical care where appropriate. Once a marketing campaign is launched, however, many just sit back and wait to see what impact their various tactics may have—or worse, just move on to the next initiative. With marketing automation, those campaigns are now only half the battle—the other half is helping to guide consumers and potential patients through to the appropriate level of engagement using personalized communications based on their behaviors. That's a big deal.

An even bigger deal is how marketing automation can be used from a clinical standpoint. Imagine that the marketing automation tactics described above lead to a patient who needs joint replacement surgery. That's marketing success, but the application of marketing automation is really just beginning. There are endless communication strategies to help patients prepare for surgery, recover from surgery, move through physical therapy, and continue to stay healthy and active for years to come. In fact, it's hard to imagine our current push for accountable care and population health management having any hope of success *without* marketing automation in the mix.

Given the dramatic impact that marketing automation could have on healthcare marketers and on the industry as a whole, it's probably not surprising that it also poses monumental challenges. For one, the technology that drives marketing automation requires integration with both CRM systems and a website's CMS. Unfortunately, many hospitals still do not have a CRM system in place and/or employ an outdated or inefficient CMS. This poses a monumental challenge for our industry, as many healthcare organizations will be unable to leverage marketing automation until they've integrated more sophisticated technology into their marketing and information architecture. (Note that a number of CRM systems companies are beginning to offer marketing automation as part of their service suite, with the biggest example being last year's purchase of ExactTarget by SalesForce. While the integration of CRM and marketing automation may seem natural, given the complex nature of both marketing technology applications, whether any CRM vendor can also excel at marketing automation will be an ongoing consideration for those looking at marketing automation solutions.)

Next, the "automation" in marketing automation often leads people to believe that the technology is essentially plug and play. That once it's in place, the dream of personalized, relevant communications is just a push of a button away. While communications are sent automatically, the development of lists, forms, scoring mechanisms, automated program flows, and other components of marketing automation can be extraordinarily complex. And every new pathway and subsequent communication created requires the development of custom content.

> Marketing automation does not replace the existing disciplines needed for successful marketing; it only enhances them.

Finally, marketing automation does not replace the existing disciplines needed for successful marketing; it only enhances them. Brand development, demand generation, content marketing, search marketing, customer relationship marketing, and all the other tools in your tool belt are still essential. To leverage marketing automation, organizations will have to expand their marketing skill set and capacity. More time will be spent planning, developing strategies, developing marketing automation programs, developing custom content, and monitoring and measuring success. Much of this incremental cost, energy, and focus will be pulled from efforts such as mass advertising that no longer hold up to the scrutiny of marketing best practices. But for many organizations, that shift will take time.

Nevertheless, marketing automation is here to stay and will usher in an incredible world of opportunities for health-care marketers who learn to embrace it. For those fortunate enough to have the leadership, systems, and know-how in place today, it can already provide a significant competitive advantage. For the rest, now is the time to start moving in that direction. So while the six key principles of developing a digital marketing mind-set that I've provided don't explicitly address marketing automation, any healthcare marketing leader who truly wants to embrace the new paradigm will eventually have to master this new strategy. And as you do, the key principles that guide the development of your digital marketing mind-set will likely change as well.

GETTING DOWN AND DIRTY

The six keys to developing a digital marketing mind-set are of course not the only principles and perspectives that may apply. Further, these six key principles are very high level in nature. At the beginning of the chapter, I used the anal-ogy of building the house to help demonstrate why becom-ing an expert in SEO will do you little good if you don't have the proper digital marketing mind-set. Unfortunately, that doesn't excuse you from understanding SEO, its value, its applications, and any of the other dozens of digital channels and tools in play today in order to master digital marketing. You will still have to climb down out of the clouds, kneel in the dirt, and get your hands dirty.

To help healthcare marketers gauge how well they are doing in building a digitally driven mind-set, Interval has created a digital marketing audit that covers a set of best practices for the *tactical* components of a smart and effective digital marketing approach.

These best practices are broken down into four main categories:

- Website
- Social media
- Value-added content
- Promotion and visibility

Each main category is in turn divided into more specific sub-sections, for a total of more than 30 best practices across the digital spectrum.

Of course, given the nature of digital marketing, what constitutes "best practices" is very fluid. So instead of providing these best practices here, where they may quickly become outmoded, we've provide the audit online at IntervalAudit. com. There, you will find these best practices along with benchmarks for each, using a scale of "leader," "average," or "lagging." Having the audit reside online allows us to ensure that we can continue to update the benchmarks as digital marketing evolves, and allows you to compare your organization against the rest of the healthcare provider industry (hospitals and health systems) and apply best practices to your marketing efforts. (Note that Interval does not distinguish or qualify benchmarks based on variables such as organization size, type, profit status, and so on because we believe that best practices should apply to all organizations, regardless of size, scope, or ability.) The online digital marketing audit is free to use and offers various levels of functionality to allow you to repeatedly benchmark your digital marketing efforts over time, among your facilities, or by various members of your team.

Like this book overall, the online digital marketing tool is based on my firm's interpretation of best practices for healthcare marketing in the healthcare provider industry. Our interpretation is based on working with clients in these areas, talking to organizations and industry experts, and continual study of recommended activities and trends in the field. The contents reflect best practices in the area of digital channels, tools, and resources applied to marketing and branding practices unique to hospitals and health systems. We strongly encourage you to visit IntervalAudit.com to take advantage of the online auditing tool and to strive for digital marketing mastery at a more tactical level.

YOUR "OH &%$#" MOMENT

At this point, you are very likely absorbing what it takes to truly have the digital marketing mind-set. If you're like most healthcare marketers, you may be having an "oh &%$#" moment. Just like the vice president in the story that opens the book, when you finally realize the depth of the change at hand and the mental rewiring it will require, you may be thinking:

- Digital needs to be a priority, something I think about all the time, not just an add-on.
- If I approach this right, eventually I won't be thinking about digital distinctly at all as a strategy.
- This is change on a scale that I may have never experienced before.

If you're having an "oh &%$#" moment, congratulations! That means you understand the scale of transformation at hand and are ready to move on to the next chapter. Just remember to have patience in developing the digital mind-set—it may take you a year or two (or more) to really get there. Keep plugging away, and keep the faith.

CHAPTER 3

THE ATTRIBUTES OF DIGITAL MARKETING MASTERY

So now you've learned the key philosophies that will help you move toward a digital marketing mind-set. Follow those guidelines, and you will find yourself on the road to digital marketing mastery. But how will you know when you've arrived?

We have developed four primary attributes that demonstrate when a healthcare marketer has achieved digital marketing mastery:

Digitally driven
Content relevant
Brand powered
Goal oriented

The attributes are supported by markers and submarkers that will help you gauge how you're doing in each of the given areas. They reflect much of what you've already read and can be used as an overall checklist to monitor your progress as you move forward. Keep in mind that each attribute represents a fundamental component of understanding and leveraging digital marketing *as it should be*. This is a critical point that deserves repeating: *These attributes reflect a future state of where a hospital or health system should be in mastering digital marketing strategies, channels, and tools.* Why the emphasis? Because these four attributes are aspirational in nature. Not just for you, but for the industry as a whole. We're not benchmarking where others are at today; we're trying to paint a picture of where you should go. Why does this matter?

Take as an example industry reports reflecting surveys of what hospitals and health systems are doing from a digital perspective. How many have mobile-optimized sites? How many use PPC advertising? How many posts do they have on Facebook each week? This type of research helps us understand the progress we're making in the industry, and can help you compare your strategies and activities to those of your peers. But this type of research has limited value because you're benchmarking yourself within an industry that is notoriously behind the curve when it comes to its level of sophistication in marketing, let alone digital marketing. This is not unlike bragging about patient satisfaction survey results that score high compared to other hospitals of similar size. How strong is your service, really, when you belong to an industry that typically ranks very low on overall service levels when compared to other industries (such as retail or hospitality)? It's like I say every time I give a Joe Public presentation: when you realize how bass-ackwards our industry has been marketing-wise, the *last* place you should benchmark your success against is your peers!

So these four attributes, and the markers and submarkers that define progress within them, have been developed to help depict a journey into uncharted territory. They were built using our understanding of the industry today, where other industries are, and where we think we ought to be going.

That means there is *plenty of room for interpretation, disagreement,* and *outright defiance.* For example, we believe that if you are exhibiting the digitally driven attribute, mass advertising will no longer be the largest part of your marketing budget. For some of you, that will be sacrilege. For others, it will be somewhat inconceivable:

"Our total budget in marketing is $5 million, and $2 million of that is for mass advertising. Nothing else comes close. How in the world will mass advertising ever not be the highest line item in our budget?"

It's definitely fair to say we have high expectations for our industry, and we know we will be pushing some folks beyond a place of comfort or understanding.

Well, that's the challenge. And as you have read up to this point, and will continue reading in this chapter, there is strong rationale behind all of these attributes. But it's definitely fair to say we have high expectations for our industry, and we know we will be pushing some folks beyond a place of comfort or understanding. The question is, will you push back, or will you use the push as energy to leap even further?

ATTRIBUTE ONE: DIGITALLY DRIVEN

Hospitals and health systems that are leading the way into the future are what we call digitally driven: digital strategies, channels, and tactics are top priorities, not supporting elements. Budgets and staff allocations, marketing plans and marketing efforts reflect an appropriate focus on "digital first"—particularly the leveraging of the web, direct, and social media channels—over mass media strategies. Marketing partners and consultants provide guidance and support based on new business models and appropriate digital emphasis, not outdated media-commission supported plans and creative.

While a digitally driven marketing discipline prioritizes digital, it also means true integration from a marketing perspective. When it comes to digital marketing, hospitals and health systems often focus on digital integration. How does social media drive engage people and lead them to your website? Do pay-per-click ads drive appropriate online conversions? What is the bounce rate for a specific page? In looking at a digital strategy, organizations typically review everything from website functionality to mobile behavior to video production... anything that can be used or shared in a digital channel or format.

Taking this mind-set further, many hospital marketing departments have positions focused on digital, including specific roles for digital marketing, social media, or websites. While these digitally focused roles are important to a successful digital marketing effort, the danger is creating one more silo that separates digital thinking from the rest of the marketing team. We have seen this frequently in relation to marketing being separated from communications, physician relations, or planning, and now we're seeing it with digital.

Just as it would be wrong to build a strategy that includes everything but digital tactics, it is equally misguided to develop a strategy that includes only digital tactics. This digital-only focus might be called an intramural strategy. When it comes to digital marketing, you should develop an "intermural" approach. Instead of focusing on digital marketing in and of itself, consider how these tools and channels will integrate with your entire marketing strategy. Sure, it's important to leverage the interconnectedness of a post on Facebook that leads to an article on your website that drives a visitor to an online health risk assessment. But it's a mistake to ignore how all of that also can be used to support your community health seminars—and vice versa—or how more people will likely access your website content when prompted by targeted direct mailings or a well-placed article in the local newspaper.

Markers of a digitally driven digital marketing discipline:

1. Digital strategies and tactics account for more than half of the overall marketing budget and are fairly represented on the marketing staff and in the external freelance/consultant mix.

> a. Mass advertising is no longer the biggest portion of the overall marketing budget.

> b. "Digital" is found throughout the marketing plan and budget rather than carved out separately from the rest of the marketing/advertising budget.

> c. Staff positions, resources, time spent, and responsibilities overall favor digitally oriented work over traditional marketing work.

2. The first priorities in any marketing effort are digitally focused (web content, SEO, SEM, social media, etc.)

    a. All significant marketing efforts rely on digital components, such as websites/web presence, SEM, SEO, content marketing, and value-added content.

    b. Mass advertising is the last path considered for most major marketing initiatives, not the first.

    c. SEO and SEM are integrated with major marketing initiatives rather than handled separately (though there may be ongoing horizontal SEO/SEM efforts independent of major campaigns or initiatives).

3. Digital managers/directors are at the table for the development of the organization's annual marketing plan.

    a. The organization's marketing plan is developed with the participation/insight of the digital team (rather than having them respond to the developed plan or not having them involved at all).

    b. One marketing plan integrates both traditional and digital strategies (rather than having a "digital" plan separate from the "marketing" plan).

4. Digital managers/directors are at the table during the development and execution of marketing initiatives (such as service-line marketing campaigns).

    a. Marketing initiatives are developed with the participation/ insight of the digital team (rather than having them respond to the developed initiative, simply execute portions ["we need a landing page"], or not be involved at all).

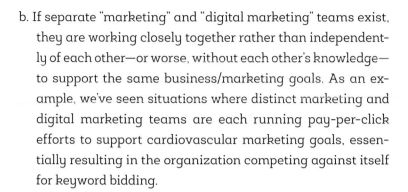

b. If separate "marketing" and "digital marketing" teams exist, they are working closely together rather than independently of each other—or worse, without each other's knowledge—to support the same business/marketing goals. As an example, we've seen situations where distinct marketing and digital marketing teams are each running pay-per-click efforts to support cardiovascular marketing goals, essentially resulting in the organization competing against itself for keyword bidding.

5. The marketing department has clear policies in place for leveraging digital marketing strategies, tools, and content for its marketing initiatives.

a. There are policies regarding the use (or limitation) of microsites and native and web apps.

b. There are policies regarding the exploration and use of new social media channels as well as for ending participation on channels that are no longer useful or irrelevant.

c. There is an organization-wide social media policy in place or being used actively.

6. Marketing leadership (traditional and digital) have established effective relationships with other functions within the organization, such as IT and finance.

a. Champions/partners/sponsors in other departments (IT, finance, compliance, etc.) have been identified.

b. Other departments are considered essential partners in effective marketing (rather than impediments or "resources").

7. When thinking digital, marketing leaders think "mobile first." That is, they consider mobile audiences as the first priority in leveraging digital channels and resources.

   a. The organization considers mobile in the context of a device rather than as a state of activity. In other words, "mobile" doesn't mean an audience member is "out and about—driving, walking, out of the home or office" but rather that he or she is accessing the Internet from a mobile device (which can happen anywhere, especially in a home or office).

   b. The organization actively monitors and updates its presence in location-based sites (Google Places, Foursquare, Yelp).

   c. The organization has or is building a responsive website.

   d. The organization uses or at least has experimented with mobile advertising.

8. Digital marketing efforts are supported by necessary technologies.

   a. A CRM system is in place and used appropriately to build communications efforts and measure results.

   b. Call center services are in place using either internal or outsourced resources to ensure efficient follow-through on marketing calls to action.

   c. Email or marketing automation technologies are in place to facilitate personalized digital communications.

   d. Electronic medical record systems allow for a robust patient portal solution.

9. Given the shift from traditional mass marketing efforts to digital, marketers must be prepared for significant and ongoing push-back from those in the organization who value old-school methods and equate effective marketing with

"visible" marketing (e.g., TV, billboards, print). To truly become digitally driven, most healthcare marketing leaders must employ change management strategies to ensure that those in the organization who have the authority to drive marketing politically will not only tolerate a shift to digital strategies but will embrace that shift. (See Chapter 8 for more on preparing the organization for the new paradigm.)

a. "Change management" is an explicit strategy expressed and pursued by marketing leadership.

b. Marketing conducts ongoing education with organizational leaders—including the C-suite, physicians, and board—to outline effective marketing efforts.

c. The organizational marketing plan is developed with a digitally driven mind-set and is presented for review and approval by organizational leaders.

d. Marketing efforts and results are regularly reported to organizational leaders.

e. Organizational champions (physicians, board members, etc.) have been identified and are regularly leveraged to help support marketing strategies.

ATTRIBUTE TWO: CONTENT RELEVANCY

Effective marketing involves creating relevant messages, content, and calls to action to targeted audiences. One of the advantages of digital marketing is that it allows for more accurate and flexible use of relevant content to specific audiences, even within the same campaign, channel, or tool. The goal is to understand the audience, the situation, and the context to deliver relevancy as effectively as possible.

One of the biggest factors behind the creation of cumbersome and confusing hospital websites is the mind-set of trying to provide information on everything to everyone, everywhere. The problem is that without prioritization of web content, everything has equal weight (particularly on the home page). So by trying to reach everyone, we instead reach no one effectively. For example, we believe in giving top priority to no more than 2–3 key audiences on a hospital's website. Content for many other audiences is obviously part of a complete site, but these audiences aren't given top priority in key areas such as the home page or primary site navigation. In addition, many hospital websites are developed in a similar way to the organizations they represent—from the inside, looking out. Audience prioritization means not only being clear about which audiences to focus on first but also designing from an audience perspective, or from the outside looking in. Effective audience prioritization maximizes relevant content for each web visitor while minimizing or eliminating irrelevant or unnecessary content and resources.

Relevancy is not just about audience but also about situational context. For example, many hospitals and health systems use popular social media channels, such as Facebook or Twitter, as promotional bullhorns, posting about their latest award or technology purchase. These posts are fine as long as they are the exception and not the rule. Facebook users are typically not on Facebook to research medical options—they're on Facebook to read up on their friends, connect with others, or check out interesting content. The fact that you've been designated a nursing magnet organization is not relevant or significant to those people—that's just chest-beating. (That may not be true of organization employees who follow your Facebook pages, but they shouldn't be your primary audience there anyway.) A great example of a lack of situational awareness comes from a long-time client LifeSource, the Minnesota-based organ procurement organization. One of its primary missions is to raise awareness of organ donation and persuade people to register to become organ donors. For years, it had set up a booth at Minnesota Vikings football games to promote this message, with a strategy of trying to be present where there were 50,000-plus people who might care about this cause. But they finally quit this promotional tactic because every time they set up their booth at a game, only a handful of people would stop by to learn about organ donation. The reason was that the situational context was all wrong—who wants to go whoop it up at an NFL game but take time out to talk about something as serious as organ donation? The situation wasn't right for the message.

Content marketing should be your dominant form of marketing altogether, not just applied to your website information architecture or social media presence. In fact, one of the best—and most difficult—ways to move beyond the old paradigm into the new is by replacing promotional campaigns with content marketing campaigns (as we'll learn in Part Two).

Markers of a content relevant digital marketing discipline:

1. The organization's website is designed to prioritize content for specific audiences.

   a. Website analytics show limited "backtracking" in visitor pathways and reduced bounce rates.

   b. Home page "real estate" focuses on no more than 2–3 key audiences (notwithstanding a footer or "universal" menu that may address more).

   c. For internal pages, especially landing pages for locations, service lines, or major initiatives, general navigation structures/content are limited, allowing for a focus on page/section-specific content. For example, when you land on the page for Cancer Services, the majority of content/navigation options you see should be dedicated exclusively to cancer and cancer services.

   d. Service-line–oriented pages contain health/wellness/preventative content and/or tools along with promotional content.

2. Content provided on social media reflects the audience and situational context of the platform:

   a. On average, more than 75% of Facebook posts (3 out of 4) are health/wellness/ educational focused or fun/activity/community focused rather than promotional in nature (promoting the services, benefits, accolades etc. of the organization).

   b. On average, more than 60% of Twitter posts (6 out of 10) are health/wellness/ educational focused or fun/activity/community focused rather than promotional in nature (promoting the services, benefits, accolades, etc. of the organization).

c. On average, more than 75% of Pinterest pins (3 out of 4) are health/wellness/ educational or fun/activity/community focused rather than promotional in nature (promoting the services, benefits, accolades, etc. of the organization). Most (if not all) pins on Pinterest should be for content with a long shelf life (think recipes, articles, tips), not short-term content such as events or promotional announcements.

3. Online advertising/promotions include a balanced/appropriate mix of promotional and content marketing–related information.

a. Ongoing pay-per-click campaigns include a mix of health/wellness/educational efforts along with efforts focused on services and/or clinical needs (rather than promotional only).

b. General consumer/patient e-newsletter/emails lead with and feature more health/wellness/educational content than promotional content.

c. Online display advertising includes a mix of health/wellness/ educational efforts along with efforts focused on services and/ or clinical needs.

d. SM advertising includes a mix of health/wellness/educational efforts along with efforts focused on services and/or clinical needs.

4. Value-added content (apps, quizzes, libraries, etc.) is used appropriately from an audience relevancy standpoint.

a. Videos include a mix of health/wellness/educational efforts along with efforts focused on services and/or clinical needs.

b. Mobile apps are developed with specific audiences in mind and appropriately targeted for use.

c. Web-based content, such as online health risk assessments, quizzes, and libraries, are developed with specific audiences in mind and appropriately targeted for use.

ATTRIBUTE THREE: BRAND-POWERED

Successful digital marketing disciplines must be brand powered. To start, it's critical to correctly define "brand." We turn to brand expert Marty Neumeier for the definition that best captures our perspective on brand:

"A brand is a person's gut feeling about a product, service or company. It's a gut feeling because we're all emotional, intuitive beings, despite our best efforts to be rational. It's a person's gut feeling, because in the end the brand is defined by individuals, not by companies, markets or the so-called general public. In other words, a brand is not what you say it is. It's what they say it is."[4]

Your brand is not your name, your logo, your advertising—it's the value your audiences give you. And in healthcare, as with many service industries, your brand is built first and foremost by what you do, not what you say. Brand value is built by the experience you deliver over time in thousands of different ways, from the expertise of your top neurosurgeon to the cleanliness of your bathrooms. Organizations that want to build a stronger brand in the market create a brand strategy, a strategic document that defines the organization's desired brand promise (or position), its brand attributes, and the ways it will embody its desired brand. The brand strategy serves as a blueprint throughout the organization for building brand, influencing priorities and decisions at all levels and across all functions.

Traditional marketing and communication strategies, such as mass advertising campaigns, are extraordinarily limited in their ability to truly build or change brand. No matter what you say, it's what you *do* that determines how audiences value you. However, many elements of digital marketing go beyond a mere communications level and actually impact consumer and patient experience in a deeper way. Digital marketing components offer healthcare marketers an opening to truly influence the user experience in ways they never could before.

A brand-powered digital marketing approach means an organization's desired brand position and attributes are reflected as much as possible in all arenas, and going further, it means digital marketing is leveraged as a way to build brand wherever possible. While your brand identity elements (name, logo, identity standards, etc.) are mere labels for your brand, their consistent and effective use is critical to clearly communicating a brand in a market. Digital marketing channels and tools can present challenges to traditional healthcare brand identity standards, but savvy marketers will adapt their standards appropriately to reflect a changing brand landscape.

Markers of a brand-powered digital marketing discipline

1. The organization's desired brand positioning/promise is reflected (if not explicitly stated) throughout digital marketing efforts. This does NOT mean use of a common descriptor or tagline in all digital arenas. Instead, it means that brand is reflected appropriately in everything from design to language to experience to tone. Examples include the following:

a. Digital marketing sophistication closely reflects the organization's desired brand position, particularly if the position or supporting attributes focus on concepts such as technology, innovation, or future. If your desired brand position reflects leading-edge technology but your website feels outdated, you're not reflecting your organization's brand position (and in fact may be counteracting it).

b. Digital marketing engagement opportunities for audiences closely reflect the organization's desired brand position, particularly if the position or supporting attributes focus on concepts such as personalized care, high touch, or community. If your brand emphasizes a caring or patient-focused experience but the calls to action on your website are all disconnected from humans (such as no opportunity to call directly or chat live online), you're not reflecting your organization's brand position (and in fact may be counteracting it).

2. The organization's brand voice—as defined by clarity of its brand message, tone, and personality—is used consistently throughout digital marketing efforts, and appropriately given distinct digital marketing venues. (Again, this does not require use of a tagline or slogan, though it could include it.)

a. Key brand messages—including the organization's desired brand position/promise and brand attributes—are used/reflected across all digital marketing efforts.

b. While brand voice is used consistently throughout digital marketing efforts, brand messaging is customized appropriately by audience. The benefits of your brand will be different—or experienced differently—for independent referring physicians than they will be for patients, for example.

c. Brand messaging is customized appropriately by channel. Language used on Facebook to talk about orthopedic offerings (a venue where the audience is not in a healthcare

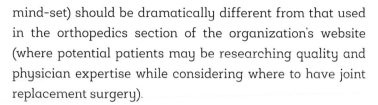

mind-set) should be dramatically different from that used in the orthopedics section of the organization's website (where potential patients may be researching quality and physician expertise while considering where to have joint replacement surgery).

d. As much as possible, content used on the website, in social media, or in content marketing efforts is proprietary rather than licensed. While a canned health library licensed from a third party is a nice supplement to a website, the generic nature of the content makes it less than desirable to use in proactive marketing efforts, such as content marketing programs or SEM campaigns. Generic content supplied from these licensed health libraries does not reflect your specific brand voice or your organization's people, weakening its power to help you build brand. In addition, canned content limits or eliminates any SEO benefits, as in many cases the content is actually hosted off-site, and/or is used by other hospitals, including potentially your own competitors.

e. The organization's brand voice is consistently applied/reflected through artwork used in digital marketing, such as illustrations, photography, video, and animations. Again, whenever possible, the organization should invest in creating its custom content to ensure alignment with brand message and voice.

3. The visual brand identity (name, logo, standards) is used consistently throughout digital marketing efforts and in a way that effectively adapts to digital marketing venues.

a. Regardless of the organization's visual identity or the digital marketing medium, the four foundational traits for corporate identity—consistency, legibility, accessibility, and professionalism—are always followed.

b. All organization websites reflect a consistent application of the organization's visual brand identity, including use of name, logo, colors, nomenclature, and artwork.

c. The organization's visual identity is appropriately displayed on websites regardless of screen size (desktop vs. mobile).

d. The organization has adapted its brand identity standards taking into consideration common requirements of social media channels. For example, you're not forcing a complex logo into a small avatar square where the text has not only become illegible but is redundant.

4. The organization takes full advantage of the ability to build/enhance the brand experience offered through digital marketing venues.

a. The organization's website provides a clean, easy-to-use, and engaging overall experience.

b. Website calls to action frequently and easily connect users to real people (call, chat).

c. The organization offers a wide variety of value-added content, such as health risk assessments, quizzes, and interactive wellness tools.

d. Social media communication includes frequent interaction with audiences (retweets, favorites, likes, +1s, responses to commenters and reviewers, etc.).

e. Digital experiences such as online classes and webinars are provided.

f. The organization leverages content marketing strategies to engage consumers in the areas of health, wellness, and prevention.

ATTRIBUTE FOUR: GOAL-ORIENTED

Leading healthcare marketers should leverage digital marketing—along with all marketing—to drive strategic business goals. That means digital efforts are derived from organizational goals and subsequent marketing goals rather than as "digital for the sake of digital" or for other unconnected, nonstrategic reasons.

In addition, digital marketing strategies should seek to drive engagement of audiences rather than simply build awareness or perception. One of the intrinsic assets of digital channels, tools, and content is that they offer the opportunity to create two-way interaction, leveraging relevant calls to action wherever appropriate. The benefits of engagement are many: Interaction creates a stronger brand impression, can lead to "actionable conversions" (changing an anonymous audience member into a known person with whom you have permission to stay connected), and helps connect marketing results to financial results (leveraging CRM systems and other methods). Organizations that leverage digital marketing efforts solely to build awareness (such as using online display advertising to "build brand") are missing the true value that digital marketing offers.

Finally, moving toward a goal requires tracking the ongoing effectiveness of your efforts. Measurement of digital marketing results is a must. Given the current climate in the healthcare industry, there may be no higher priority for healthcare marketers today than dedication to measuring marketing results. Healthcare reform, shrinking reimbursements, consumerism, increased and new forms of competition, new business models—all of these market forces are fundamentally changing our industry. And part of that change is an increased pressure on provider financials—there are no two ways about it. That means more pressure on marketers. Most marketers constantly battle to defend their budgets, their departments, and sometimes even their own positions. Many deal with organizational leaders—CEOs, CFOs, physicians—who often have little or no concept of how marketing truly works or how it benefits the organization. As financial pressure on the healthcare industry continues to mount, the pressure on marketers to prove the worth of their efforts will also continue to increase. When it comes to justifying the value of your marketing efforts, the best defense is a strong offense—it's up to you to drive how marketing success is defined.

The good news is that digital marketing channels, tools, and resources lend themselves extraordinarily well to measurement. The bad news is that many healthcare marketers are unsure of how best to measure digital marketing effectiveness. In some cases, marketers are unfamiliar with the various methods of measurement or with which metrics matter most. In other cases, they are overwhelmed by the sheer quantity of data that digital marketing efforts can produce. Most often, digital marketing efforts are not tied to strategic marketing goals, let alone business goals, making any attempt at measuring effectiveness somewhat of a moot point. No matter how deep or broad they may measure, leading marketers constantly try to tie digital metrics back to strategic business objectives.

Markers of a goal-oriented digital marketing discipline:

1. Digital efforts are initiated, developed, and managed in correlation with strategic marketing goals and objectives.

   a. Most digital efforts originate from a business/marketing planning process rather than being pursued from a reactive position.

   b. Digital efforts and their related budget and staff allocations are prioritized according to strategic business/marketing goals.

   c. The marketing/business purpose of digital efforts is easily discerned, and the organization avoids launching new efforts just for the sake of going digital. For example, the development of a native app that shows emergency room wait times (a tool very few consumers would value enough to download and store on their mobile device) could be considered "digital for digital's sake."

2. Digital marketing measurement is appropriately utilized and acted upon.

   a. Website analytics are reviewed regularly.

   b. Social media analytics are reviewed regularly.

   c. SEM analytics are reviewed regularly.

   d. SEO ranking for key service areas and key terms/phrases is reviewed on a regular basis.

3. Digital marketing measurement is appropriately prioritized (not "data rich, information poor").

   a. Key performance indicators (KPIs) are tracked.

   b. Reports are produced with prioritization and analysis of key metrics.

4. Systems and processes are in place to tie digital marketing results to business goals.

    a. Calls to action that lead to actionable conversions are prioritized.

    b. Unique URLs, phone numbers, and other customized tools are used to tie specific digital marketing efforts to specific results.

    c. Processes/responsibilities are in place to connect marketing conversions to patient utilization.

    d. A CRM system is in place and appropriately used to connect actionable conversions to patient utilization.

    e. Key relationships in finance and IT have been made to connect marketing conversions to patient utilization.

5. Digital marketing results are reported regularly, transparently, and in a way that connects to marketing and business goals.

    a. A dashboard is used to report results tied to strategic goals.

    b. Metrics are tied to patient utilization and marketing ROI whenever possible.

    c. Reporting allows for deeper dives where appropriate/necessary.

    d. Reporting goes beyond basic metrics, such as Facebook likes or website visitors.

    e. Reporting is available to everyone internally on an ongoing basis (rather than restricted to certain audiences at certain times).

CHAPTER 4

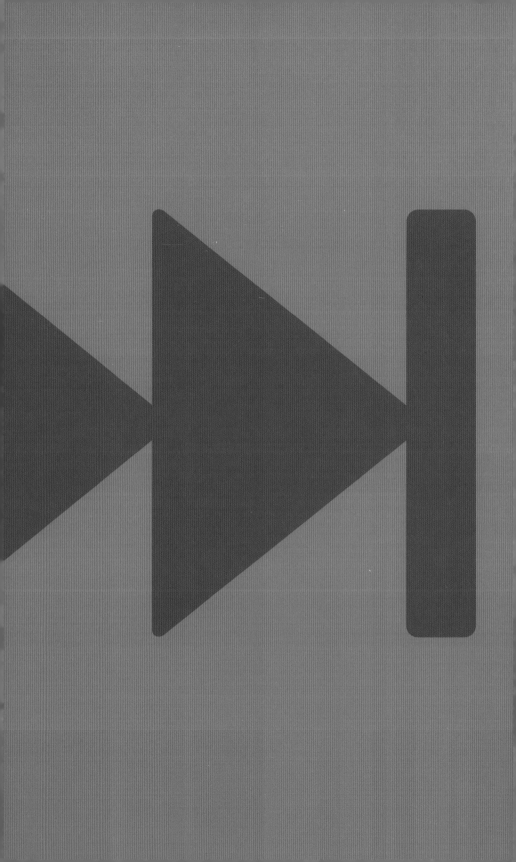

CASE STUDY: DIGITAL TRANSFORMATION

If you're not at least a little overwhelmed after reading this section on mastering digital marketing, then either I haven't done my job well enough or you have ice water running through your veins. There's no getting around the idea that mastering digital marketing to make the move to the new consumer healthcare marketing paradigm is a monumental endeavor. But imagine you could find someone who could help you make it happen. Someone you could helicopter in to help you find your way to the new paradigm, to help you build the digital marketing mind-set, to help you not only establish the right strategic vision but also leverage all the digital marketing channels, tools, and resources in an effective fashion. That person might look a lot like Chris Boyer.

Chris has been asked to help build digital marketing mastery at not one but two health systems. His experience is extensive, and he is a recognized digital marketing leader in the industry, speaking at conferences across the country. The bad news is you won't be able to hire the actual Chris Boyer into your system. The good news is you don't have to. As Chris himself would tell you, anyone with the curiosity and drive to master digital marketing can make it happen. And more good news—Chris is more than happy to share his experiences with anyone who's interested. So while you can't bring Chris himself in, you can learn from his story of how he's moving his current organization forward.

THE CHANGE AGENT

Chris started his digital transformation work at Inova Health, a seven-hospital system in the Washington DC market, where he spent four years helping the organization move from the old paradigm to the new and moved to the position of senior director of digital marketing. He built a robust social media program. He helped create one of the most celebrated and successful digital marketing programs, FitFor50 (which also happened to be an early poster child for content marketing). He introduced SEM, SEO, and other digital marketing disciplines, and he and his team created one of the first fully responsive health system websites, inova.org.

In 2012, Chris moved to North Shore-LIJ Health System, a massive health system based in the greater New York City area, that consists of 17 hospitals, 400 ambulatory and physician practices, and a service area of more than seven million people. While his title changed (he is associate vice president, digital marketing at North Shore), his charge didn't: bring the system into the new paradigm with a focus on digital marketing mastery.

"In my first interview, they made it very clear: they wanted to bring digital to the forefront but weren't sure how," he said. "My purpose was to help bring the concept of 'digital first' to their marketing efforts."

THE STATE OF THE DIGITAL STATE

His first step was gauging the existing digital marketing situation. What he found was not surprising and fits the profile of most hospitals and health systems across the country in terms of digital mastery:

- The organization was pursuing digital marketing but in a very fragmented way. Digital was certainly a secondary thought, not "initial and integrated."

- The system's website was overgrown, disorganized, and poorly designed, with non-actionable and text-heavy content and an outdated and expensive content management system. It was also not built using responsive design and thus not optimized for mobile audiences (even though 45% of the site's traffic came from mobile devices).

- The initial audit uncovered 40 different microsites in use at North Shore, and since that time, more than 40 others have been discovered. While microsites themselves aren't necessarily a bad thing, the microsites at North Shore-LIJ had not grown out of a strategic effort but instead had been allowed to sprout willy-nilly across the system. As a result, most were poorly designed and didn't follow the system's brand guidelines, and the sheer quantity made it nearly impossible to adequately manage them all.

- Search engine marketing was being performed, as Chris puts it, "for digital's sake," with budgets assigned to large pay-per-click advertising campaigns that led to ineffective landing pages, in one case with no call to action whatsoever. (A lack of click-through activity from a Google AdWords pay-per-click campaign can hurt an organization's quality score, which can lead to higher costs for keywords.) Search engine optimization practices weren't even the responsibility of the internal digital team. Instead, an outside vendor was "optimizing" web content using outdated and sometimes harmful practices.

- Social media, which was (and still is) managed by the public relations staff, had no input or influence from the digital marketing team.

- The CRM system was underutilized. Few marketing efforts were being measured using CRM, data was not being updated appropriately, and use of CRM was not aligned with the organization's strategic planning.

- The organization had dabbled in email marketing, but only in isolated efforts with very little tie-back to marketing strategy.

- The digital marketing team operated in its own silo within the marketing department, which was perhaps the biggest reason for the low level of digital marketing efficacy.

As occurs in many organizations, the state of affairs at North Shore-LIJ when Chris arrived was not created intentionally; it was more the organic result of decades of living in the old paradigm.

Digital was always secondary and separate, always at the end of the line,

"Digital was always secondary and separate, always at the end of the line," says Chris. "A classic example is with landing pages for large campaigns. The request for a landing page always seemed to come just a week or so before the campaign was supposed to launch in the market. I can't tell you how many times this happened. We even had instances where marketing folks would build a landing-page URL into the advertising and have everything ready to go without checking first with the digital folks to see if the URL was even available to use."

SETTING A COURSE

As the famous saying goes, admitting you have a problem is half the battle, and hiring Chris into a position that hadn't existed before was a clear indication of the organization's desire to fix the digital marketing problem. To help set the right tone for the transformation and to set a clear vision for how to move forward, Chris's next step was to create a 100-day plan. The plan had two primary purposes: First, it painted an honest picture of the current state based on the initial audit, showing how far behind the organization was in terms of best practices for digital marketing. Second, the plan presented a future state for how Chris and his team would help close the gaps and move the organization to digital marketing mastery. The future state included a digital vision, key goals and objectives, measures of success, target audiences, and more.

"There were of course lots of operational changes that needed to be made in order to leverage digital marketing more effectively," says Chris. "But from my viewpoint, the biggest challenge ahead of us was moving the digital team to a position of leadership in the marketing organization. We would need to build our bench strength in order to handle all of the new responsibilities, and we would need to figure out how move upriver in the process to ensure digital was treated as a strategic component of our marketing efforts, not an afterthought."

One of the primary ways Chris accomplished this was by creating a new role, "digital strategist."

THE DIGITAL STRATEGIST

While Chris made many changes in terms of how the digital team operated, perhaps the most important was the creation of the digital strategist role. As occurs with most healthcare marketing leaders, he was restricted in his ability to add head count. There were positions to fill, surely, but the bigger challenge was ensuring that digital had an appropriate place at the marketing table. That was the primary purpose of the digital strategist designation, which wasn't a new position but instead was a title given to those leaders on the digital marketing team who could help bridge the gap with the rest of the marketing organization.

"Bringing on a digital marketing leader at the level of vice president helped demonstrate the organization's desire to advance digital marketing, but I couldn't be everywhere all the time," says Chris. "Those who served as digital strategists would play the role of advocate for digital marketing wherever it was needed. These are people who understand how digital marketing can be applied in a business setting AND who understand how to drive marketing goals."

As written in the original 100-day plan, digital strategists had the following attributes and responsibilities:

- Meet with business lines, physicians, and marketing to understand business goals and objectives
- Focus on equal collaboration with marketing manager

- Have broad understanding of digital platforms and how they could be applied

- Create digital marketing strategy document

- Coordinate digital marketing team resources to deliver on strategy

- Use measurement to determine success and improvement

- Provide regular updates on digital marketing strategy to clients

- Create executive-level briefings—present to upper management

A digital strategist was assigned to each area of marketing, public relations and other lines of business, including community health and the foundation. The digital strategists would work hand in hand with the primary marketing lead in any marketing effort. The purpose was to ensure that digital marketing was effectively leveraged by having a digital strategist at all meetings to provide insight and guidance and to help manage expectations from internal clients ("we need a new website for our clinic by Monday!").

Not surprisingly, the idea of introducing digital strategists into the existing marketing process caused some concern. Would the addition of another marketing representative confuse internal clients, undermine the marketing lead, or slow the marketing process?

"This was all about relationship building, and we had to demonstrate that the inclusion of a digital strategist in the process wasn't a threat but a resource for the marketing lead," says Chris. "It required constant communication between the marketing lead and the digital strategist, and it had to be founded on trust."

Chris says that in the first year of this new setup, there were definitely challenges and some push back. But now digital strategists are seen as invaluable resources to the marketing team, which has helped the organization overall make huge gains toward mastering digital marketing.

"The marketing lead and digital strategist are now locked arm-in-arm as a team," says Chris. "In some cases, the marketing lead will let the digital strategist contribute the digital marketing component of a marketing plan. In other cases, we're even seeing 'digital osmosis,' where the marketing leads are learning from the digital strategists in a way that allows them to more effectively leverage digital marketing themselves."

(Remember the snake eating its tail from the beginning of Chapter 2? Having traditional marketing professionals become digital experts is a perfect example of that. At some point, the marketing leads won't need digital specialists at the table because they *will* be digital specialists themselves.)

THE TRANSFORMATION CONTINUES

The introduction of digital strategists along with other changes under Chris's watch have helped North Shore-LIJ make significant strides toward digital marketing mastery. SEO and SEM practices have been upgraded, social media activity has become more collaborative within various marketing strategies internally, the organization is exploring the use of marketing automation, and a massive effort is underway to redesign the organization's website and upgrade its dysfunctional content management system. The process is fairly straightforward: Assess the situation, map out a vision and plan, make the necessary change internally, and execute. But there's nothing simple about it—the transformation can take years. At North Shore, although much as been accomplished, there's still a tremendous amount of work to be done. But as Chris Boyer has shown (twice), it can be done.

PART TWO

CONTENT MARKETING MASTERY

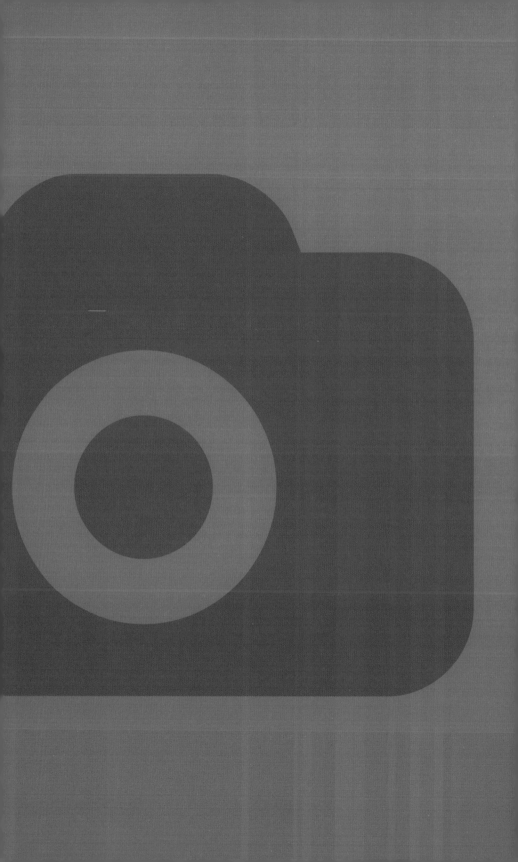

CHAPTER 5

OUR SELFIE PROBLEM

In Chapter 2, I used my "Jerry Maguire" memo to the healthcare industry to help tear down one part of the existing consumer healthcare marketing paradigm: mass advertising. Now let's use a popular phenomenon in today's culture—the selfie—to expose the other part of the paradigm: promotional messages and content.

The "selfie"—the self-directed photo style that has come to dominate many social media channels, particularly among the teenage set—has caused a lot of handwringing among social commentators. For many, it represents the further plunge into self-absorption that the Millennial generation has been associated with for a number of years (fair or not, the stereotype is widely applied to anyone under 30 years of age).

Personally, I don't mind the selfie. I've taken many selfies in my life, even before the advent of the two-camera smartphone made them so easy to take, and, subsequently, so common. I can remember back in college taking selfies with old-school cameras. Thanks to my long arms, I developed quite a skill for pulling off the selfie, which came in handy when my buddies and I wanted to have some fun with the disposable cameras that were often set out at weddings.

But what if every photo you took was a selfie? Or even if most of them were? What if your family photo album was full of pictures of you mugging for the camera rather than of the people you love or the places you've been?

As silly as that might seem, that's pretty much the case with hospital marketing. The idea of the selfie as a metaphor (or is it analogy?) for one of our industry's major marketing problems hit me as I spoke to a large group of financial and legal folks at the 2014 HFMA Region 11 Healthcare Symposium in San Diego in January 2014. As I have done many times over the past few years, I was giving a version of my *Joe Public Doesn't Care About Your Hospital* keynote, which includes a rant on how we waste millions of dollars every year delivering chest-pounding, promotional messages to a public that mostly doesn't need our services and, therefore, doesn't care how awesome we are.

What if every photo you took was a selfie?

The vast majority of my presentations are to healthcare marketers, but that day I was trying to explain this concept to folks who don't have a background in marketing. And as I was laying it out, it hit me: "You know what these ads are? They are selfies! Billboard-sized selfies, and they are the dominant form of marketing in the hospital industry." The audience laughed and smiled and nodded—they got it. Not only the analogy (or is it metaphor?) but the import of the comparison.

As I always say when I promote a shift from the old paradigm to the new, that doesn't mean you will never run a billboard again. Instead of being the first-out-of-the-gate, knee-jerk response to every marketing challenge, promotional mass advertising should be the last item on your list, given its inordinate expense and lack of impact on our targeted audiences. As with selfies, one or two isn't bad. You just don't want every image you present to say "look at me—I'm awesome!"

THE SHIFT TO CONTENT MARKETING

Incredibly enough, the phrase "content marketing" appears nowhere in the first Joe Public book. Oh, the concept is in there, and is, of course, the focus of the first chapter, which reflects the name of the book. But rather than calling it "content marketing," I referred to it with its synonymous label, "inbound marketing." Here's a snippet:

> According to the HubSpot Inbound Internet Marketing blog, inbound marketing is defined as "marketing focused on getting found by customers." It is the opposite of traditional, or "outbound marketing," with its goal of "finding customers." (Or what Seth Godin calls "interruption marketing.") In this model, instead of pushing your message out to potential customers to compel them to try your product or service, you create content of one kind or another that pulls people in and makes them want to find out about you. Instead of running

TV commercials, it's posting videos people want to share on YouTube. Instead of a print ad, it's a blog. In a way, it's the difference between quantity and quality. With outbound marketing, the quantity of impact is usually measured, and more is always better. (Think of the millions of impressions you might get from a mass advertising campaign.) With inbound marketing, your goal is far fewer contacts, but those contacts are of much higher quality because they want to connect with you. So while the numbers may be lower, the effort is more effective because you've spent far less money for more qualified contacts.

Since that time, the term "content marketing" has sprung up everywhere in healthcare—online forums, industry articles, conference keynotes. But the meaning is the same no matter what you call it. Of course, providing relevant content and messaging to audiences seems obvious. The goal is to understand the audience, the situation, and the context to deliver relevancy as effectively as possible. Yet if that's the case, why do we struggle so mightily with the concept in healthcare?

THE CONTENT MARKETING MIND-SET

As with digital marketing, to master content marketing in healthcare, you need to develop a certain mind-set. *Unlike* with digital marketing, the premise for that mind-set is extraordinarily simple and straightforward. The *application* of that mind-set, however, is more nuanced.

First, what do we mean by content marketing? Most hospitals and health systems are already employing some level of content marketing. Your online health library? That video on how to ease back pain? The healthy cooking article in the community newsletter? The joint pain seminar at the public library? The online heart disease risk assessment? All of these are good examples of content marketing in action. (Remember, not all content marketing tactics are digital.)

There are many definitions of content marketing floating around. For us, **content marketing is defined as the strategy of targeting audiences with messages, information, tools, or interactions that have value to the recipient outside of a purchasing need**. Messages and information regarding your organization may be included, but if they are, they are secondary. This differs from promotional marketing, which is focused solely on touting your benefits and/or selling your services, or even touting your brand as a whole. In short, content marketing is about them, not about you.

In healthcare, you can use content marketing to connect with consumers in many ways, whether by providing health and wellness resources, entertaining audiences, or even connecting with stories that are relatable to the audience in question. A simple example of the difference: If you run an ad promoting your joint replacement surgery center, that's promotional marketing. If you run an ad that provides tips on how to treat knee pain after jogging, that's content marketing. Of course, in the end, you want to connect those audience members to your service when it's appropriate. We are still talking marketing, after all.

There are many reasons that healthcare organizations should leverage content marketing, but the primary reason is that the vast majority of people in your market—Joe Public—don't need your services today, next week, or even next year, rendering promotional efforts about your service lines, physicians, or offerings very ineffective.

MOVING FROM SCATTERSHOT TO STRATEGIC

While the idea behind content marketing—using non-sales messages and content instead of promotional messages and content—is simple enough, things get a little more complicated from there. How does content strategy play into all of this? And does content marketing itself need to be further defined?

To help further refine the concept of content marketing, let's once again apply the idea of horizontal and vertical thinking. On the following page you'll find a horizontal/vertical model applied to content marketing.

Notice the horizontal activities that are related to content marketing, such as posting community events on Facebook or developing a brand journalism offering. Remember that horizontal activities are those that take place on a continuous basis, regardless of what your current marketing priorities, goals, or campaigns are. As mentioned earlier, most hospitals and health systems today are conducting some type of horizontal content marketing effort, whether they call it that (or realize it) or not. In fact, providing nonpromotional content is something that has been going on for decades.

While it's admirable to use content marketing in any way, the vast majority of organizations rely strictly on horizontal activities, and typically in a scattered, supporting, or secondary fashion. The online health library? Buried on your website, impossible to pull forward and leverage in smart ways. The video on back pain? A one-off that is nowhere to be found in your latest orthopedic advertising campaign. Your online heart disease risk assessment? Some don't even allow you to capture user metrics or information.

To boost the impact of horizontal content marketing efforts, you need to develop and implement a *content strategy*—a plan that ensures you are leveraging content in the most effective way possible, applied to a specific use. There are different types of content strategies, depending on what the content strategy is meant to support. For example, you could create a content strategy to guide horizontal content marketing across the organization, which would typically be delivered through platforms such as social media. Or, you could create a content strategy for your website, which would guide the development and ongoing maintenance of copy, artwork, videos, tools, and other types of content on your website. Even within content marketing, there are different applications for a content strategy. For example, one subset of content marketing is brand journalism, which itself has many definitions. But for hospitals and health systems, brand journalism is typically done in an effort to develop a "WebMD"-like resource for medical content that can be used by the media or consumers. Given its unique structure and purpose, a brand journalism effort might have a different content strategy than other content marketing efforts.

So now that I've cleared that up (?), how important is content marketing and the use of content strategies to your marketing effort? Very important. How relevant is it to the new paradigm? Not necessarily relevant at all. That's because while leveraging content marketing in a horizontal fashion is smart, it's not really a huge departure from what you may

(continued on page 118)

VERTICAL

Advanced
- Extended marketing automation ——————
- Multi-channel advertising ——————

Outreach
- Enhanced social media efforts ——————
- Custom SEM efforts ——————

Basics
- Heart health risk assessment ——————
- Extended content ——————
- Responsive landing pages ——————
- Themed campaign ——————

HORIZONTAL

- Brand journalism ——————
- Marketing automation ——————
- Classes/events ——————
- Social media ——————
- Content strategy ——————

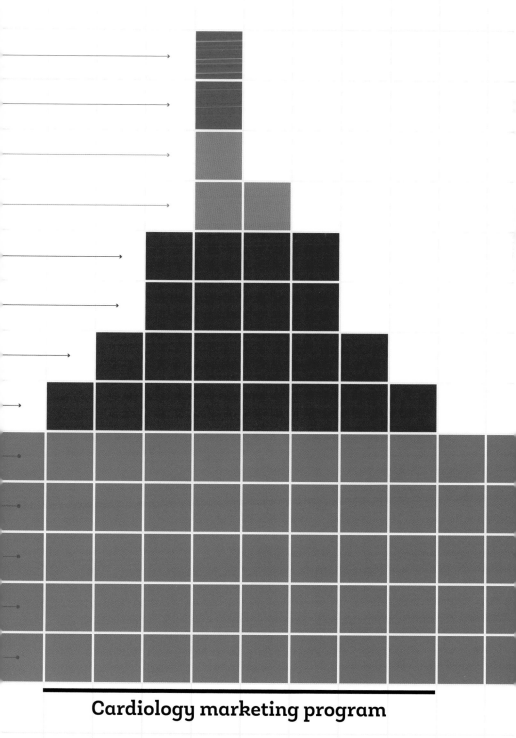

Horizontal & Vertical Efforts

Content Marketing

Cardiology marketing program

be doing now. It's just a gradually more sophisticated, more effective application of the discipline.

But we're not after gradual. We're after a wall-smashing, canyon-jumping *paradigm shift*. That means we want to go *vertical* with content marketing.

> We're after a wall-smashing, canyon-jumping paradigm shift.

I encourage you to learn more about horizontal content marketing applications, particularly through social media and other digital efforts, and how to properly build and implement content strategies where needed. We won't cover that here. There are already fantastic books dedicated to these efforts, and there's little I could add to the mix (to start, pick up Ahava Liebtag's *The Digital Crown* to learn all you need to know about developing a content strategy). In the next chapter, we will explore how to go vertical with content marketing to once and for all change our selfie habits.

CHAPTER 6

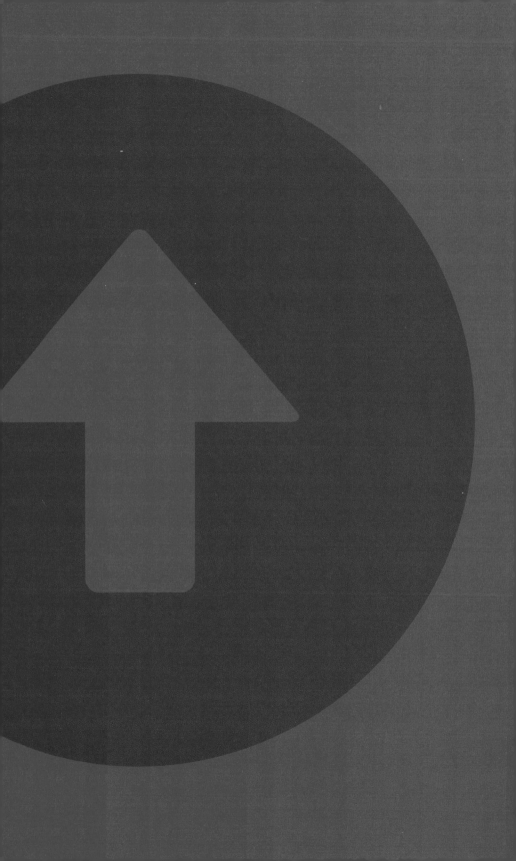

GOING VERTICAL WITH CONTENT MARKETING

Remember, the premise behind the content marketing mind-set is simple enough—replace "promotional" messages and content with "non-sales" messages and content. "Joint pain" instead of "joint replacement surgery." "Warning signs of eating disorders in teenagers" instead of "world-class eating disorder clinic." "Health" instead of "ambulatory surgical center." As I alluded to in the introduction to the book, however, the fact that this difference is easy to understand doesn't make it easy to implement. In fact, the irony is that although achieving digital marketing mastery involves a far more complex transition, for many healthcare marketers, it will be easier to achieve than attaining content marketing mastery. That's because even the most backward-thinking, uneducated (from a marketing-standpoint), and opinionated doctor understands at some level the need to progress technology-wise to adapt to social media, the web, or mobile. Replacing promotional messages with content messages, however, is not an intuitive evolution. Again, *horizontal* approaches to content marketing pose no real threat to the old-school way of thinking.

"You want to create a video on how to avoid back pain? What's the harm in that? You want to post heart healthy recipes on Facebook? Go to town!"

It's when you want to achieve true transformation by taking content marketing vertical that you will feel the pain.

"You want to replace our six-month, $3-million television campaign promoting our five-star surgeons with a content marketing program? Say again?! What are you smoking?!"

In our industry, moving away from promotional advertising campaigns is not only utterly contrarian to what most people believe is effective, but it's counter to what they see all around them from other hospitals and health systems. If I'm a CEO or orthopedic service line director or chief cardiovascular surgeon, all I see, everywhere I look, is "We're five stars this" and "We care that." Why in the world should we go away from telling everybody how awesome we are, *especially when it comes to achieving our most important marketing goals?* That's why real marketing transformation comes from going **vertical** with content marketing, which simply means replacing promotional campaigns to solve your marketing challenges with content marketing programs. Recall the horizontal/vertical depiction of content marketing from the prior chapter.

Are you being asked to support the cardiology service-line growth goals? To help a new physician build her practice?

To "build the organization's brand"? Instead of addressing vertical challenges such as these with a promotional mass advertising campaign, you will connect with more people and drive greater (and more easily measured) marketing results with a content marketing program. *That's* how you really move the needle. *That's* what I mean by going vertical with content marketing.

SO WHAT'S THE DIFFERENCE?

How do you go about moving away from relying on promotional advertising campaigns to leveraging content marketing programs? Your initial step is actually the same as it's always been. You begin with the same questions you would have when facing any strategic marketing challenge:

- What are our goals? our business goals? our communications goals?
- Who is our target audience(s)?
- What are the measures of success?
- How are we different in this area from our competitors?

Once you have a fundamental understanding of what you want to accomplish and whom you need to target, you're ready to take a different path toward a solution. Rather than focus on a campaign based on promotional messages, mass advertising, and selling your services, your focus is on developing a program based on educational messaging and content. You're also setting out to create something that's more sustainable—that's why we use the language of content marketing *programs* in contrast to promotional *campaigns*. A campaign, at least in its typical promotional advertising form in healthcare, typically has a set shelf life of 6 to 12 months. Some last longer, some are shorter, but they are intended to end when they are deemed no longer "fresh" in the market. That's because campaigns rely primarily on a creative theme or hook to give them weight and get them noticed, and that hook loses steam over time. There are certainly exceptions to this, with hospital promotional campaigns that have lasted years. But typically, campaigns are intended to have a lifespan measured in months, not years.

A *program* is different in two key ways. For one, it is typically multifaceted. It's not just about communicating a message; it includes experiences, activities, tools, or other ways consumers can engage. But in addition, a program should be designed to last *years*—at least a couple, but hopefully more. While it can take more effort and resources to create, once a content marketing program has been created, the content itself will have legs. That series of videos you create will have value for a long time. And although you will still need to add content to keep the effort fresh over time, it won't require a complete retooling of the message, theme, or creative approach.

The chart that follows helps to clearly demonstrate the differences between a promotional campaign and a content marketing program as a strategic solution to your marketing challenge.

Traditional promotional campaign VS Content marketing program

Traditional promotional campaign		Content marketing program
Sales/promotional	**Typical message**	Non-promotional (educational, health/wellness)
Mass advertising	**Primary channel**	Digital
PR, microsite, landing pages, direct marketing	**Secondary channels**	Event or experience, PR, direct marketing
Creative concept	**Primary differentiator**	Value, depth, packaging of content
Promotional copy, artwork, video	**Type of content**	Educational copy, tools, video, events
Potential focus of creative concept	**Role of clinician**	Content sources, supporter of content
6-12 months	**Typical shelf life**	2-3 years
Awareness, perception, web analytics	**Primary measurement**	Conversions, Event attendance, ROI via CRM
Easy to do, valued by organization, high profile	**Pros**	Stronger brand building, relevant to broad audience, engage along continuum, sustainable marketing, more/better metrics
Expensive, ineffective, difficult to measure, real target audience is tiny	**Cons**	More legwork, not understood by organization, ongoing content required

As the chart shows, you will likely use digital channels as the primary means to engage your audiences, though you certainly can leverage face-to-face, print, and other mediums as well. This is why it's important to separate digital marketing mastery from content marketing mastery. There is significant overlap, but not all digital marketing takes shape as nonpromotional content marketing. For example, a pay-per-click campaign on Google may target those seeking joint replacement surgery, a purely *sales-oriented* challenge. Likewise, not all content marketing takes digital form. Some of the most powerful content marketing, for example, takes place with live experiences, such as a class, seminar, or community event.

You will still need to ensure that your program is both compelling to your audiences and differentiated from all the other hospital marketing noise in the market. So you'll still need creative packaging, but rather than creative applied to an advertising campaign, you'll need creative that ties together the entire program—the web experience, content, social media integration, and any promotional tactics. But we'll talk about that more a little later in the chapter.

CONNECTING CONTENT MARKETING TO BUSINESS GOALS

Now that you have a general idea of what it looks like to go vertical with content marketing, let's make sure you're able to articulate and demonstrate the value of a content marketing program within the organization. After all, if I'm claiming that content marketing programs are superior to promotional campaigns in most instances, I need to back that claim.

Be ready to have to hit a higher standard for proving the worth of content marketing as a strategy, at least early on. One of the most frustrating aspects of content marketing in healthcare is what we call the "old vs. new double standard." For years, hospitals and health systems have spent millions of dollars on promotional mass advertising efforts, often with little or no results tied to actual business goals such as market share, volumes, physician visits, or marketing return on investment (ROI) that shows the direct financial contribution of marketing efforts to the bottom line.

> Where was the demand for business results when the organization spent $1 million on a six-week TV campaign promoting its five-star award?

Yet when marketers push for more effective and less costly content marketing strategies, suddenly there is demand for proof of results. This pressure often comes from C-suite executives, but sometimes even from senior marketers who are less familiar with content marketing, digital, and newer marketing strategies.

"Yes, I see how we've tripled traffic to our website, but what do those click-throughs really mean? Until we can prove this supports our business objectives, let's put these efforts on hold."

Where was the demand for business results when the organization spent $1 million on a six-week TV campaign promoting its five-star award? While this double standard may be frustrating, here's the good news: It's exactly what you want to hear. The inherent nature of content marketing will help you prove why it's far more effective at driving business results than your chest-pounding ads ever were or will be.

ENGAGEMENT IS THE SECRET SAUCE

Promotional marketing often casts a wide net, hoping to reach those people who have a clinical need today. There may be a prompt to call, to visit a website for more information, or to schedule an appointment. But the vast majority of those hit by such a message do not need a doctor or hospital and therefore have nothing to respond to. With this much larger group, the hope (a false hope, I'd say, given that Joe doesn't care) is to influence audience attitudes by increasing awareness, perception, or mindshare.

With content marketing, you should always strive to move beyond measuring success in terms of impressions, awareness, or perception. Because you're providing relevant messaging and content to potential patients *and* consumers, you can focus on driving actions unrelated to seeing a doctor or scheduling a surgery. In other words, you're striving for *engagement*. Yes, just as with digital marketing, the lifeblood of content marketing measurement is engagement. Your audiences aren't just going to hear your message and hopefully change their opinion; they are going to take action from your effort, one way or the other. When you engage your audiences, you can demonstrate the effectiveness of your marketing in many ways, ultimately tying your efforts back to clinical utilization and the bottom line.

How do you entice your audiences to take action? That depends largely on whom you're targeting. Most content marketing programs, regardless of focus, message, or market, have two primary audiences: those seeking care (prospects) and those seeking health information and resources (healthcare consumers).

You may prioritize those audiences differently depending on your effort, but you should always strive to accommodate both audiences with any content marketing effort. Of course, you would like to drive in patients today, so the first audience is essential. But the ultimate value of content marketing is its appeal to those who don't need your services today but may tomorrow. This is a much, much larger audience and critical to your future success, making consumers just as important as prospective patients.

As we will discuss a little later, your content marketing program message, theme, and content can have 1,001 different angles. In this section, we're focusing on tying your efforts back to business goals, so we will focus solely on calls to action that will help you measure results. As you review the calls to action that follow, realize they may be leveraged in any number of ways through social media, advertising, educational materials, within marketing automation programs, and, most importantly, in your content marketing program's web presence.

ENGAGING PROSPECTIVE PATIENTS

For those in the market who are looking for your services, the goal is to help them move to the next relevant step in their care as quickly as possible. There are numerous calls to action to help with that goal, and they are similar to what you've likely used in the past with more traditional promotional efforts. They include the following:

"Schedule an appointment"—using a phone number, email form, or chat

"Ask an expert"—allowing prospective patients to submit questions about their situation, often to clinical staff

"Request information"—providing literature or other informational pieces regarding the service or ailment in question

"Take a tour"—depending on the situation (maternity care, for example); prospective patients may find this of value

Remember, this audience has a clinical issue and is actively searching for a solution. Your content marketing program may have drawn their interest with educational information or creative packaging, but people from this audience are looking for clinical help.

It's important to make sure that whenever these audiences are ready to reach out and seek help from you directly, the calls to action—particularly on your program's web presence—are easy to find. And as with any marketing effort, make sure you are using customized calls to action, such as unique phone numbers or URL tags, so you can more directly connect website traffic to your marketing efforts.

ENGAGING HEALTH CONSUMERS

Although patient acquisition is always your ultimate marketing goal, the vast majority of consumers are not in the market for your services. However, there are many people in your community seeking to improve their health in one way or another. Some may have risk factors they want to learn how to manage. Many others are looking for information and tools to help them lead a healthier life. While these consumers don't have a problem requiring a doctor or hospital today, they represent a much larger audience full of potential future patients. You likely already have numerous programs and services aimed at this healthy population. Content marketing then becomes an extension of those efforts.

Your goals with this audience are twofold: One, you want to provide actions aimed at those who actually *may* need clinical care today but don't realize it and move them to the first audience group, prospective patients. Two, you want to engage the rest by providing actions that allow you to stay connected with them until they need clinical care down the road.

Common calls to action for this audience may include the following:

- Screenings
- Online risk assessments
- Community seminars
- Interactive health/wellness content and tools
- Specialized native apps or web apps
- Webinars
- Live tweeting, tweet chats, and hangouts
- "Ask an expert" functions
- Newsletters (printed/electronic)
- Affinity programs
- Support groups

Although you want to drive consumers through to clinical care when appropriate, your goal with many of these actions is simply to connect with those who don't need your services today but may down the road. The more engaged consumers are, the more likely they are to remember you when the time comes that they actually need healthcare services.

PULLING IT ALL TOGETHER

The engagement opportunities listed here combine with other marketing metrics to help paint an overall picture of how your program is faring. There are generally two levels of metrics you want to build:

Aggregate level

This is where you rely on metrics that demonstrate overall engagement with your program, which will help you determine what parts of your program are working effectively, how different promotional efforts (such as a kick-off event or PR push) change activity, and how to compare these efforts to others of a similar nature. Metrics at the aggregate level can include the following:

- Web analytics
  - How many unique visitors did the program generate?
  - How many visitors came to the program's web presence directly, through organic search, or through inbound links?
  - What was the bounce rate for this traffic?
  - How long are they staying?
  - What content are they spending time on?

- Online marketing conversions
  - What is your click-through rate for online ads (search or banner)?
  - What is your cost per click?
  - What percentage of visitors take the desired action step?

- Overall action metrics
  - How many people called the information line?
  - How many people requested an appointment?
  - How many people watched a video?
  - How many people attended a community seminar?

This is a short list, yet look at all of that data you can measure tied directly to your marketing efforts!

Even at this level, you can correlate your marketing efforts to business success. For example, if you've increased traffic to the oncology section of your website fivefold through a six-month content marketing program and physician visits increased 15% in that time, you have a strong case for how your marketing is driving business.

Individual level

While the aggregate level of measurement should provide a wealth of information regarding the success of your marketing effort, tying your content marketing program to business results requires going to the individual level. That is, how are actual individuals being pulled through the acquisition funnel by your content marketing efforts and engaging your organization with reimbursable services? Tracking this requires some form of CRM system.

As you are integrating calls to action throughout your content marketing program, your ultimate goal is the actionable conversion. We've defined this before, but as a refresher: By **conversion**, we mean you've turned an unknown visitor to your website or an unnamed attendee at your joint pain seminar to a known individual. Because he or she has taken a specific action, such as requesting information, registering for a webinar, or taking an online risk assessment, you know the person's name, contact information, and possibly more. By **actionable**, we mean you've collected this information in a way that, with the individual's permission, allows you to take action with him or her specifically. Maybe you can follow up on a poor risk-assessment score with a phone call. Maybe you can send an e-newsletter. Maybe you can invite the person to a community seminar.

> The actionable conversion is needed to continue marketing to the individual in relevant ways.

The actionable conversion is needed to continue marketing to the individual in relevant ways. This requires relationship marketing, which is often forgotten in the focus to launch a marketing initiative. All that effort and money spent to connect with a healthcare consumer, yet no plan for how to stay connected moving forward? A good rule of thumb is that you spend as much time planning strategic relationship marketing as you do planning the content marketing program itself. And, as alluded to earlier, leveraging marketing automation technology will bring your relationship marketing efforts to new heights. (But that's fodder for another book.)

But just as important as its role in relationship marketing, actionable conversion allows you to track the individual against clinical utilization. Using CRM, you can track those who have engaged your content marketing program in your patient information file, which allows you to track patient utilization. Using ROI calculations, this in turn will allow you to determine exactly how much money your marketing effort is bringing the organization. This process can be very complex, of course, and requires a CRM system, which itself is a significant investment. However, these are the business results your leaders will care about the most. (For more information on calculating marketing ROI, pick up *A Marketer's Guide to ROI* by David Marlowe[5].)

In the end, some of the metrics and processes outlined here could be used with old-school mass campaigns promoting your services just as they can be used for content marketing efforts. But the differences are significant. Because your efforts will be relevant to far more people, your overall success will be greater. And because of the nature of content marketing programs, you will have far more opportunity to measure your results and prove the true business value of your marketing strategies.

WHEN CONTENT MARKETING IS EVERYWHERE, HOW DO YOU STAND OUT?

Content marketing is the new "It girl" in marketing circles. Everywhere you turn—blog posts, seminar presentations, "gurus," newsletters—content marketing is the hot topic. While healthcare is traditionally slower in adopting new marketing trends, the cat is most likely out of the bag for hospitals and health systems, so first-mover advantage is very likely gone in your market. That makes it even more important to build your content marketing program in a unique and compelling way.

It gets worse. Not only are your peers shifting their gaze to content marketing, but it seems every other company in every other industry is aiming for the healthcare consumer. When you leverage health and wellness from a content marketing standpoint, you're no longer just competing with other hospitals and health systems for the consumer's attention. You are competing with the likes of Nike, General Mills, and Walgreens and with technology such as FitBit, Basis, and Jawbone. You are also competing with mobile apps such as LoseIt, MyFitnessPal, or HealthTap. Some of these products come from individuals and companies that lead the world in design, innovation, and consumer branding, and they are often supported by monster budgets. Heck, even a wine store in Minneapolis runs an annual "heart healthy" wine sale. How can you compete with that?

Despite these challenges, content marketing is still one of the best strategies for hospital and health system marketers to build brands and drive business. You just have to develop strong, differentiated programs.

You have something they don't have

When it comes to competing for the attention of healthcare consumers with non-provider organizations such as Nike or apps such as LoseIt, you have an asset they don't have: a position in the consumer's mind as the leading source of medical expertise. Whether you're a two-physician practice or a 20-hospital system, most consumers believe that when it comes to understanding health, wellness, and medical issues, doctors, nurses, and other caregivers "know best." According to a recent survey from the National Research Corporation, when asked to rate their trust in various audiences, 74% of consumers rated doctors and nurses as "highly trusted." That was the highest ranking of all audiences listed, followed by hospitals at 68%. Fitness and health companies were far down the list at 27%, with insurers right behind at 26%.

Your goal is to bring that expertise front and center by leveraging not only your doctors but all manner of clinical experts. Don't forget the other brilliant minds you have on staff, such as nurses, nutritionists, physical therapists, and PAs. You want to know the best way to include your docs in your marketing? Forget the picture of your orthopedists with their arms crossed and the headline "Outstanding in our field." *Show* how outstanding they are by demonstrating their expertise through videos, articles, community seminars and appearances, social media interaction, and other content or engagement-centered tactics. Thus, you are no longer *telling* consumers about your expertise; you are actually *demonstrating* it. Use your built-in advantage—your clinical expertise—as the foundation for your content marketing program.

Make it your own

To begin lifting your program above the fray, it's important to make it your own. Every organization has a unique brand, and your program should reflect your organization's brand.

Here are some ways to draw that out:
Create your own content—there are any number of great resources available to license online health and wellness content, from social media fodder to canned blog posts to entire

medical libraries. The problem with licensed content is that it's not *your* content. That means many other hospitals— even potentially one right down the street—may be leveraging the exact same content. Not only does that make differentiating that content impossible, but it drains the power of search engine optimization to pull folks in. While it requires effort and resources, you're better off creating your own online content that reflects your brand voice, your clinical expertise and opinions, and your expert providers.

Remember, healthcare is local. While it's true that this adage is changing somewhat (medical tourism, anyone?), for the most part, people are still driven to seek out care close to home for the majority of their healthcare needs. There are reams of helpful medical information on WebMD, but what do I do with it once I've found it? Who can help me? Whom do I talk to if I want to do more or schedule a visit? Build your proximity advantage into your content marketing program. Include community events and seminars. Partner with local businesses to build healthy offerings, or fitness centers to create branded programs. Work with local celebrities. Develop an interactive map that highlights resources in the community related to your program. Focus your search engine marketing efforts on tying content to your locations. It may be impossible to compete with WebMD or other massive health information sites when it comes to natural or paid search for terms such as "Alzheimer's disease." However, you can add your location to that search term, as in "Alzheimer's disease in Minneapolis," to break through and become findable for those searching.

Highlight your competitive differentiation. Depending on the focus of your content marketing program, you likely have any number of advantages over your local competition. Let's say your program is supporting an orthopedic marketing effort. If you have the best joint replacement center in town, be sure to include seminars there. If you have the most orthopedists on staff, reflect that by featuring as many as possible in videos or community events. Figure out what your brand strengths are and thread them through your content marketing program.

Package your program

Search Google for "back pain," and thousands of results come back. Clearly, it's not enough to just put out quality content. You may be able to provide a better level of content than non-healthcare companies, but that will do little to separate you from your peers. Earlier, we drew a clear distinction between content marketing programs and traditional promotional campaigns. But in one way they are the same—creative packaging can help drive differentiation in the market and draw audiences in. Here are some tips to help achieve that: Make it interesting—go beyond the obvious of healthy recipes, blog posts, and educational videos. Include a strategic mix of online tools, gamification, events, and other engagement-oriented tactics to bring your program to life. In many cases, given the nature of content marketing, you'll have the opportunity to make your program fun, which can be difficult in more traditional hospital marketing efforts.

Find your program's *raison d'etre*—your program will be more successful in engaging your targeted audiences if it's based on some sort of motivator for your audience. This motivation will provide a reason for folks to engage and serves as a foundation for your entire program. Here are some examples: (For more on these examples, visit thinkinterval.com).

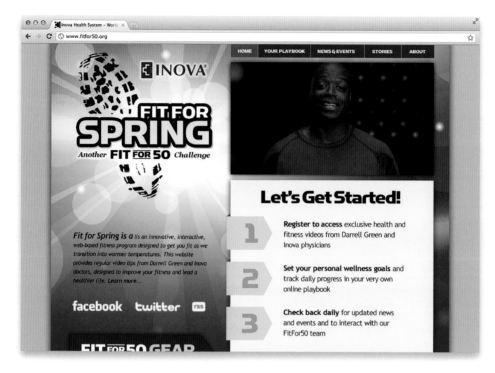

Many people want to become healthier but don't have a way to formulate a plan. The "Fit for 50" program at Inova Health System, which ran from 2009 through 2013, encouraged people to develop their own 50-day fitness program, providing an easy, accessible means for participants to improve their health.

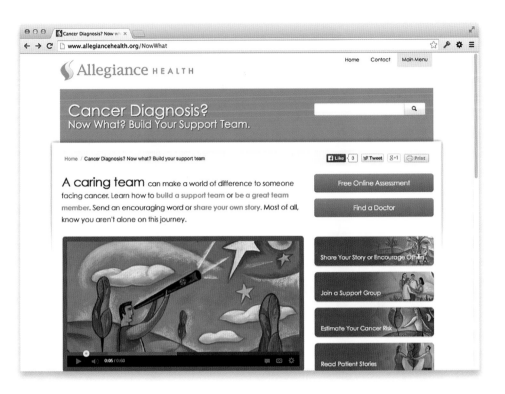

People dealing with cancer often face the unknown and don't know where to turn. The "Now What?" program for Allegiance Health provides answers to the difficult questions people face all along the continuum of cancer, from worrying about family history to finding an odd lump to facing a diagnosis.

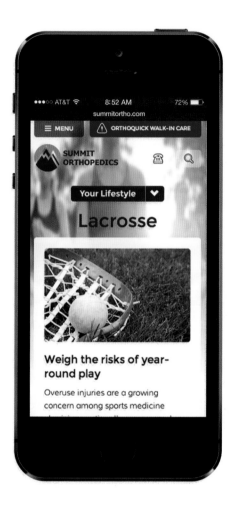

If you're looking to stay healthy and avoid injury while exercising or participating in sports, you're looking for simple, relevant advice. The online QUICKGuides from Summit Orthopedics provides snappy, easy-to-access content, including QUICKTips and videos in the general topical areas of fitness, recreational sport, parenting, outdoor activity, and everyday life.

OVERCOMING OBSTACLES

In Chapter 8, I provide overall advice on how to prepare the organization for moving from the old paradigm to the new. But there are some challenges specific to going vertical with content marketing that are helpful to understand at the outset.

Watch out for the "volume alarm"

In our early work with clients to develop content marketing programs, many efforts never made it to market. The marketing leader believed in content marketing as a strategy, and money, time, and effort were invested in building a compelling program. But the program failed to launch because someone in the organization had pulled the "volume alarm."

What's the volume alarm? First, hidden in the administrative offices of health systems across the country, I imagine a volume alarm installed in the wall that looks like a fire alarm but instead reads as follows:

"Pull only in the case of extreme concern about stagnant or declining volumes. Must be pulled at least twice per year, preferably more often."

Even in today's age of reform, hospitals and health systems still need increasing volumes, and likely will always need certain levels of volumes to stay viable. (While reform in the form of accountable care and population health management is supposed to help keep people out of the hospital, we don't *really* want to keep everyone out of the hospital.) So in every organization, there is a constant monitoring of census and volume goals, and inevitably, alarm bells go off at least a couple of times per year. Typically, those are related to a fiscal year that's winding down, a key quarterly report that's been issued, or some other event that causes C-suite concern about volumes.

When that happens, the content marketing program you are developing is likely to come under attack. The problem is that it can take some time to go vertical with a content marketing program and create something with differentiating value in the market—just as it takes time to create a massive promotional advertising campaign. That means it's very likely that at some point during the development process, someone will pull the volume alarm in the organization, which will lead to declarations such as this:

"While I'm onboard with the idea of content marketing, we need volumes NOW! So let's shelf that effort and get ourselves back out in the market and drive in patients with our billboard campaign touting our award-winning service."

The problem here, of course, is the assumption that an award-winning service billboard will drive in patients (which it won't), while a content marketing program won't drive in patients (which it will). Old-school advertising campaigns survive the volume alarm because people mistakenly think they help drive in volumes. But the volume alarm is a content marketing program killer. And here's the thing— you will always experience volume alarms, which can make it very difficult to see a content marketing program through to launch.

Be smart—anticipate this dynamic and get out ahead of it. Continually reinforce the idea that content marketing programs are *designed* to not only drive volumes but to do so more effectively than promotional advertising campaigns. Get out ahead of the volume alarm and be prepared. Reiterate your current marketing strategies, revisit your marketing plan, reinforce how you've gained success through similar efforts in the past. Also be strong in the face of volume alarm-induced panic. Acknowledge the panic, acknowledge the need for volumes, and convey that you have things covered.

Shift your thinking on resource allocation

One of the most common refrains we hear from marketers who want to pursue content marketing and then see a full-blown content marketing program concept is this: "Wow, that's a lot of content. That's a lot of work. We don't have the time/resources/focus to do all of that."

It's definitely true that a content marketing program takes more labor to create than a promotional advertising campaign. A strong program concept typically includes the need for compelling, differentiated content—articles, videos, apps, events—which take time and resources to create. Most hospitals and health systems do not have the staff resources to create all of that content—thus the anxiety.

A shift in thinking regarding resource allocation is required to embrace going vertical with content marketing. Remember, we're replacing a typical promotional mass advertising campaign with a content marketing program. For years, we've had no problem spending thousands if not millions of dollars on creating gigantor television, outdoor, and print campaigns. How do we pull off marketing efforts of this scale with our understaffed marketing departments? Well, we outsource it, of course. We pay agencies to create campaign concepts, execute all the elements, and buy and place the media.

If you're thinking your staff can't create and execute a content marketing program all by itself, you're not comparing apples to apples when it comes to resource allocation. If you're replacing a giant advertising campaign with a content marketing program, you have $100,000, $500,000, or $1 million at your disposal. Let's say you had a budget of $1 million for a one-year mass advertising campaign promoting your orthopedic service line, which would cover creative development, ad production, and media planning and placement. Instead, you're going to create a robust content marketing program.

For starters, it's important to remember a key tenet of content marketing when compared to promotional marketing: You should expect to achieve the same results for far less money with a content marketing effort, or achieve far greater results with the same budget. That's true first and foremost because content marketing—especially combined with digital marketing efforts—reaches far more people with relevant information, thus driving more engagement and patient/consumer action than promotional advertising. Second, while promotional advertising has demonstrated an impact only while it's still in the market, the content from your content marketing program will provide value long after you stop promoting its existence. As long as it's available online, people can search for it and find it, and you can point audiences to it through social media. And finally, you won't have to pay so much money to publicize your content marketing program because the content itself provides value to your audiences, which means they will be far more likely to share the content themselves.

So back to that budget of $1 million. Let's take one quarter of that and allocate it to content development. Imagine the articles, videos, app, events, and other experiences, online or other, that you could develop for $250,000 through outside agencies, consultants, and freelancers. That would be some incredible content—more than plenty to create a compelling content program. And you still have $750,000 left, which you *could* use for promotional efforts (even including mass advertising!), for a higher-level online experience, or for more events. Or you could minimize your media spend, relying primarily on social media and search to drive traffic, and pocket the rest.

Don't completely abandon promotional advertising

Because taking content marketing vertical and replacing your standard advertising campaigns can seem like such a dramatic shift to those you serve in the organization, don't start off with an "either/or" approach. You can assuage a lot of anxiety from service-line leaders, C-suiters, and physicians if you still produce some level of promotional advertising. The difference will be limiting your efforts and expenses in this area. Instead of a full campaign, create a series of print ads. Instead of hyper-expensive television, produce some far cheaper radio spots.

The truth is, you will never abandon promotional advertising, nor should you. There are certainly times when promotional advertising makes sense—when introducing a new service, for example, or opening a new location. Building awareness in those instances is a laudable goal. Even when content marketing makes more sense, save a little for promotional advertising to help grease the skids internally. It will take time before the rest of the organization catches up and understands the value of the new consumer healthcare marketing paradigm. Rather than continually knock heads, make life easier on yourself by allowing for that transition.

CHAPTER 7

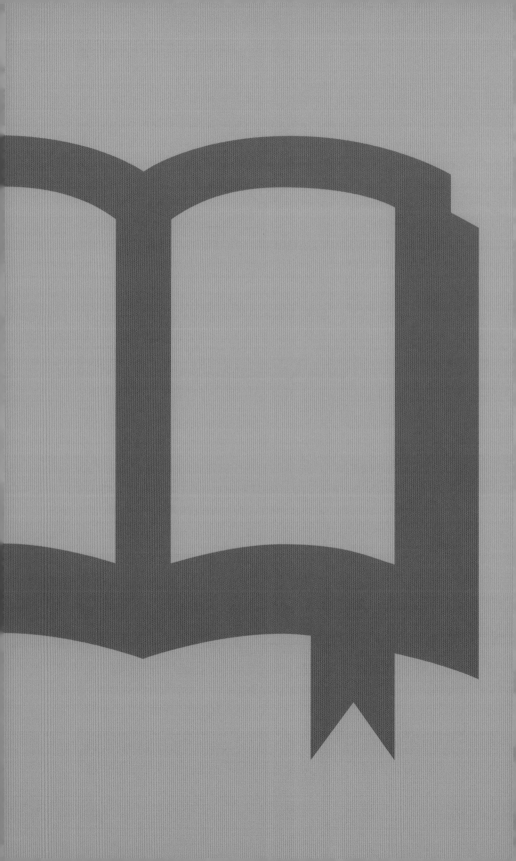

CASE STUDY: THE STORY OF THE STORIES

As I note in Chapter 6, examples of content marketing can be found at virtually every hospital, clinic, and system in the land. Educational videos, community classes, and health fairs have been around for decades. What *isn't* easy to find are examples of organizations that have truly gone vertical with content marketing, replacing the giant promotional campaign with a similar-sized content marketing program. We've provided a few on our firm's website, but one of the best examples I've come across of a full-blown, honest-to-goodness content marketing effort gone vertical is the "Stories of the Girls" program from Advocate Health Care in Chicago.

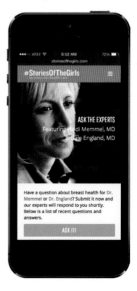

Softening the ground

For Advocate, the inspiration for this content marketing effort supporting breast health awareness and their breast cancer service line came from another expanding application of content marketing—brand journalism. According to Christine Priester, vice president of marketing at Advocate, the organization's brand journalism effort, dubbed "Health enews," was instrumental in paving the way for something bolder.

"Health enews was our first really conscious effort to stop talking about us and instead provide those we serve with information and resources that were about them," she said. "The incredible success we had with the effort—there are now more than 200,000 subscribers to 'Health enews' since its inception in 2013—helped prove that this philosophy had merit. We began thinking 'we can do this with everything.'"

The first opportunity to apply the philosophy of content marketing to a service-line marketing effort came with the organization's breast cancer services. But even with the brand journalism effort's success, which helped to mentally prepare organizational leaders for more content marketing, Priester says the marketing team knew this was something altogether different.

"Breast health was really the perfect opportunity, because there is so much about women and their breasts that we could talk about," she says. "But this was our first foray into a strategic, service-line oriented content marketing program, and we had no idea how it would work. Or if it would work."

The resulting "Stories of the Girls" program was, in Priester's words, "the most successful campaign we've ever done." The program's theme is to create and facilitate the conversation around women and their breasts—primarily from a health standpoint, not just a cancer-prevention/management perspective. Here's how the program is introduced on its website:

"From training bras to weddings, breast health is more than an exam or diagnosis. It's the essence of womanhood. It's the lifelong relationship you have with your breasts. It's the conversation taking place right here and now."

The focus of the program is its website, www.storiesofthe-girls.com, which helps facilitate that conversation through a number of venues and provides a comprehensive level of content and tools related to breasts, breast health, and breast cancer. Where appropriate, it connects women to services offered by Advocate, including opportunities to connect with clinical experts and schedule a mammogram. What about this program made it so successful?

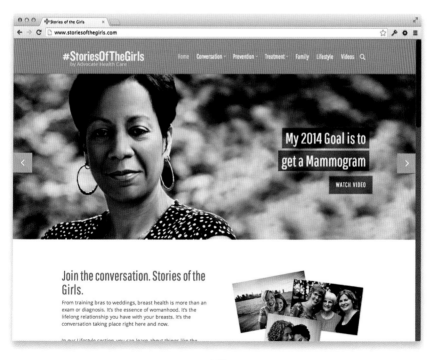

Packaging counts

Like any content marketing program, "Stories of the Girls" prioritizes information and resources that are not about touting a service or the organization itself but about helping women with their questions and issues involving their breasts. This includes providing educational information and videos on breast health, a three-step plan for preventative care, an online "Ask an Expert" service, community events, compelling stories, support groups, counseling sessions, and more. In fact, your organization may offer some or all of these types of resources itself. But as we learned in Chapter 7, it takes more than just providing valued content to go *vertical* with content marketing. Take, for example, the program's *raison d'etre*—spurring conversation among women about their breasts, a conversation that most women are having at some level among their friends and family members. Providing a central theme gives the program and its message focus, which helps consumers understand *why* they should pay attention.

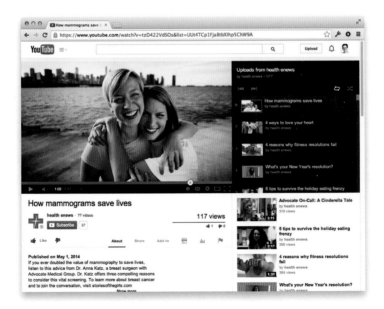

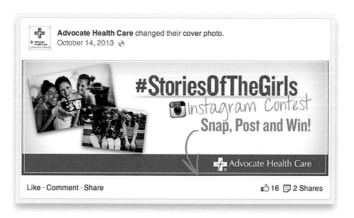

"We wanted this to be about more than just breast cancer; we wanted it to be about a huge part of every woman's life— their boobs!" says Priester. "Women talk about that all the time. Of course, they don't call them 'breasts' though."

That, of course, points to another aspect of this program that reflects one of the keys to content marketing success— creative packaging. As I've mentioned earlier, content marketing will attract more people because it provides something of value to more people than your promotional messages, but to go vertical with a content marketing program, you still have to package your effort in a differentiating and compelling way. And boy, does this program offer creative differentiation. This isn't a program about breast health; this is a program about the stories of the "girls," a popular euphemism for breasts that women use. Content and communications surrounding the program don't shy away from the topic of the "girls," either, with one video featuring a 60-something woman smiling as she holds up a giant fuchsia bra, and another featuring a trio of preteen girls singing, "We must, we must, we must increase our bust!" All of this makes the program seem real and accessible, not phony or corporate. And as with all strong creative, it evokes strong feelings, both positive and negative.

Not surprisingly, the campaign has elicited some strong reactions, says Priester. For example here's a quote from one email the organization received: "I do not refer to my breast as 'the girls.' I feel that it is distasteful to hold up a huge pink bra in the pictures. Embarrassing!"

By far, however, the responses were overwhelmingly positive, says Priester.

"We received so many messages—from breast cancer survivors and just women overall—thanking us for being brave enough to tackle these issues in a human, realistic way."

Bringing the program to life

As noted earlier, the organization's previous foray into brand journalism helped pave the way for going vertical with a breast health content marketing program. That doesn't mean the idea didn't meet with resistance internally, says Priester. She adds that the organization's chief marketing officer, Kelly Jo Golson, was instrumental in helping move the idea through the organization.

"We knew we wanted to go down a content marketing path about a year before the program was actually launched, and we knew that this type of effort would require a different level of engagement with internal audiences," says Priester. "Kelly Jo essentially did a road show, advocating this decidedly edgy approach with clinical leaders, site presidents, and others. We knew there would be a select few who would hate it, but overwhelmingly people internally loved it, especially the women. Even our most opinionated clinical 'marketing experts' were on board."

Although Priester says they still received the occasional old-school push back—"Where's the message about our breast center accreditation?" or "We're not telling them about ourselves!"—being able to point to the success of the Health enews brand journalism effort really helped to assuage any fears.

While "Stories of the Girls" fits the prototype of a smart vertical content marketing effort in so many ways, the most important reflection of success is that it surpassed its marketing and business goals. This is critical, given the common perception by many non-marketers that while content marketing may seem nice or "feel good," only promotional messages and campaigns drive business. (My perspective, of course, is that it's actually the opposite.)

The program, which was promoted in the Chicago market from mid-September 2013 through early November 2013, resulted in a 10% lift in mammographies throughout the system, a key metric of success for the effort.

"We're not sure whether this was better or worse than a promotional campaign because this is so new to us and we don't yet have that apples-to-apples comparison," says Priester. "But in all ways that we measured results, this was a success. And that doesn't even include an ROI calculation of downstream utilization, because we're still building our CRM systems. Of course that's where so much of the success comes from any health, wellness, or prevention-focused campaign."

In true new-paradigm fashion, although Advocate did use limited mass advertising in the form of limited television, outdoor, and print advertising, these channels were em-

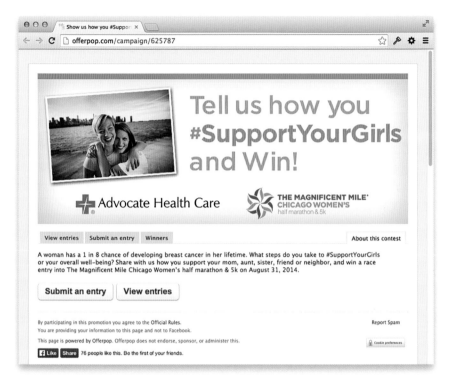

ployed only in support of what Priester calls a "huge" digital push, which included a robust, *responsive* program website, significant social media outreach, search engine marketing, and local and national online display advertising.

Beyond the increase in mammographies at Advocate, the program delivered in many other ways during its three-month promotional window, including the following:

- More than 800 calls to the "HealthAdvisor" call center

- A nearly 15% increase in Health *enews* subscribers

- More than 45,000 unique visitors to the program website

- Increased social media followers and engagement

The program is still getting results, says Priester, as the online content and events that support the program live on even after mass promotion of the campaign in the market ended. For example, the program has generated more than 3,300 calls, 1,200 web requests and 1,100 appointments through May 2014, eight months after its inception. As I noted earlier, this is a huge advantage of a content marketing program over a traditional promotional campaign, where the impact (which is limited to start with, given its irrelevance to such a vast majority of consumers) is typically felt only while promotional messages are running. The content developed when you go vertical with your effort has legs well beyond any paid promotion. As long as you're able to continue supporting your effort with a strong web presence and even just social media outreach, your program will pull in your audience. And as long as your content lives online, people will be able to search for it and connect with it. If your program is strong enough, it

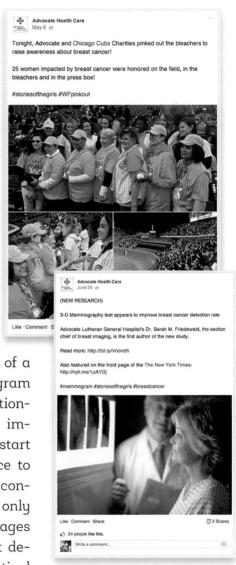

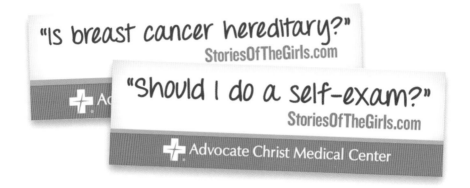

will also gain earned media far beyond what a promotional campaign could hope for. For example, the NBA's Chicago Bulls found the "Stories of the Girls" so compelling that they invited cancer survivors featured in the effort to be honorary captains at a Bulls' game during Breast Cancer Month. The program has been deemed so successful that the organization is gearing up for a renewed effort—"Stories of the Girls 2.0"—launching in September 2014.

With its clear theme, strong creative, wealth of content and experiences, and tremendous results, the "Stories of the Girls" effort is really the poster child for going vertical with content marketing. It represents what happens when you cross into the new consumer healthcare marketing paradigm and provide true value to audiences with your marketing efforts.

PART THREE

BRINGING IT HOME

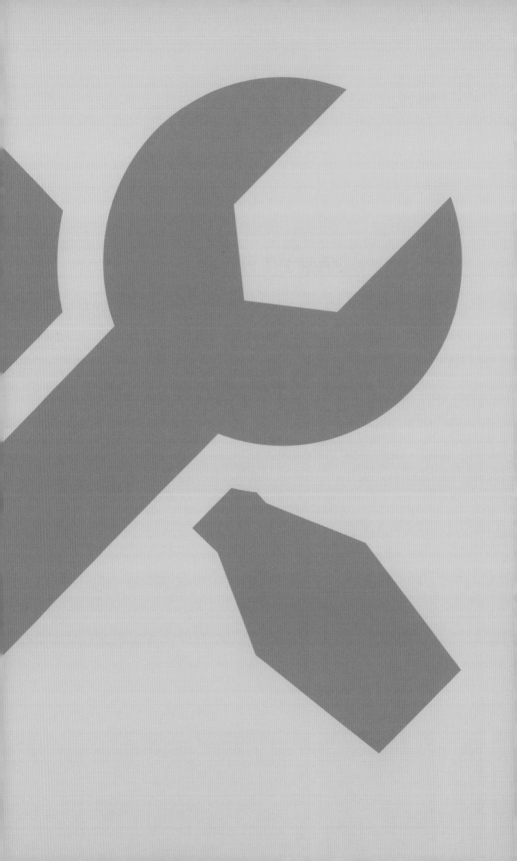

CHAPTER 8

PREPARING THE ORGANIZATION FOR THE NEW PARADIGM

How challenging is a paradigm shift? In 1962, Thomas Kuhn wrote *The Structure of Scientific Revolution*, introducing the idea of paradigm shift. He stated that scientific advancement is not evolutionary but rather is a "series of peaceful interludes punctuated by intellectually violent revolutions," and in those revolutions "one conceptual worldview is replaced by another."[6]

> A paradigm shift is a series of peaceful interludes punctuated by intellectually violent revolutions.

Many paradigm shifts of the past were not only "intellectually violent" but actually violent. Remember in the introduction, I noted that Copernicus didn't reveal his sun-centered-universe theory until his deathbed for fear of persecution? Galileo's support of "heliocentrism" led to years of house arrest. His predecessor, Italian friar and philosopher

Giordano Bruno, was actually tried for heresy and burned at the stake at the Italian Inquisition in part for believing that even the sun wasn't at the center of the universe.[7]

Thankfully, no blood has been spilled (to date) in the pursuit of the new consumer healthcare marketing paradigm. But as a paradigm shift, it is definitely a very difficult transition for hospitals and health systems. After all, the old paradigm still dominates our industry. Those who support our marketing efforts—advertising agencies and media buyers, for example—have business models built to thrive on the huge production expenses and mass media commissions that are native to traditional mass advertising campaigns. As marketers, we know how to create old-school campaigns—we know who to hire, we know the process, we know what to expect. Creating multimillion-dollar advertising campaigns is easy compared to mastering digital marketing or convincing our organization to embrace content marketing. Not only that, but it's fun, and that sparkling television spot looks amazing in our portfolio. And perhaps most important of all, not only will we not get fired for producing promotional mass advertising campaigns, but we will often be celebrated as heroes throughout our organization for finally getting the word out and taking it to the competition.

So it's easy to see why the vast majority of hospitals and health systems are still stuck in the old paradigm—those responsible for marketing can't, won't, or don't know how to move forward. Those who do want to move forward face nearly insurmountable odds in many cases. Our leadership, our physicians, our organizations, our industry—all are aligned against the paradigm shift. How can we help them see the light so we can do what's right?

Given the scale of shift from old paradigm to new, it is not enough to just believe in the transformation yourself. You must find ways to move others within the organization past the all-too-common addiction to the old paradigm or risk having your efforts devalued, disrupted, and unsupported. Marketers wanting transformation must approach content marketing from the perspective of true organizational change. How do you make that happen?

Illustrate how "visibility" no longer equals "strong marketing"

You've probably heard something like this more than a few times in your healthcare marketing travels:

"I saw our billboard today—great job, marketing!"
or, more likely, this:

"I see our competitors out in the market, but not us. We need better marketing!"

These oft-repeated statements in all their variant forms represent a mind-set tied to the old paradigm: *Strong marketing means we're visible. If we're not visible, we must be weak in marketing.* This of course made sense when there was no Internet, no mobile phones, no social media, no search engines. When the primary forms of communication were mass media channels such as television, radio, outdoor, and print.

Just as we need to move away from those dinosaurs to more effective marketing strategies and channels, we also need to retire the idea that marketing equals visibility. Think about it—in the new paradigm, many of your marketing efforts will be *invisible* to those in the organization making that judgment call. For example, the only way to "see" your robust search engine marketing efforts is to search for the right keyword on Google. Not only would a CEO have to think to take that step to "see" what marketing is up to, but he or she would have to understand all the work that has gone on behind the scenes to make that effective. And to top it off, a billboard is 50 feet high and bathed in spotlights, while a pay-per-click ad is a text blurb in the corner of a web page consisting of a total of 130 *characters*.

This is one of those dynamics that can be addressed logically but really hits certain people in an emotional place. "I don't care how effective SEO is; I want to see our name in lights!" So make sure you continually reinforce why visibility no longer equates to effective marketing; why if the CEO isn't seeing your marketing, that means she probably wasn't targeted by it; and that placing your emphasis on connecting with people where they are through SEM, SEO, email, and other digital tactics is what smart marketing is all about.

Use heavy appliances

When I speak at conferences about the concept of *Joe Public Doesn't Care About Your Hospital*, I use a technique I call the refrigerator exercise to help demonstrate that if you're not in the market for a product or service, you don't care about that product or service (thus rendering promotional mass advertising ineffective and leaving digital and content marketing preferable alternatives for reaching consumers). What's great about the refrigerator exercise is that it's one you can easily perform with those in your organization. To start, ask if the person or audience has bought a refrigerator in the past couple of years. If so, you'll need another type of low-interest product or service, such as a law firm or life insurance company—companies or products that most con-sumers need only a few times in a lifetime. Then the conver-sation goes something like this:

"First, can you list the top-selling refrigerator brands? OK, that's a pretty easy one. Most folks can name at least a few. What about the top-selling models? Or what are the differ-ent types of refrigerators available? Now, let me ask, which manufacturer is known for making the best of each type of refrigerator? Which refrigerator model or brand is rated the highest by consumer reports? Which brand is known for having the most state-of-the-art refrigeration technology? What, by the way, are the latest cutting-edge refrigeration technologies? At what price points will you find refrigera-tors? Who makes the highest-priced refrigerators, and who is known for offering the best value in refrigerators? What colors are available? Finishings? Ice-making functionality? Produce-drawer innovations? Can you tell me which refrig-erator brand was recently named the five-star award win-ner for manufacturing quality by the American Association of Refrigerator Manufacturers?" (That last one is made up, but that's kind of the point.)

At this point, people will start to get the idea. A select few may actually be able to answer some of those questions. Perhaps they just moved into a new home or renovated their old one and had to shop around for a new refrigerator. Per-haps their trusty icebox finally quit working after all these years, and it was time for a replacement. But 95% of us don't know anything about refrigerators because we don't need a refrigerator, and we haven't had to shop for one for years (if ever). And because we don't need one, we don't know much about them and don't take time to learn about them. Basically, we don't care about them. And there, ladies and gentlemen, using refrigerators as our analogy, lies the certain but painful truth: Because the majority of consumers don't need a hospital, physician, or health system at any given time, they don't care about those services.

Using this exercise helps bring home the idea that promotional hospital marketing is irrelevant to the vast majority of consumers. Only by embracing relevant messages and content (such as health and wellness delivered as a content marketing strategy) can you hope to connect with consumers who are not actively seeking the services you're selling. At the same time, the excercise helps support why digital marketing efforts, such as SEO, SEM, and well-designed, responsive websites, are the most efficient way to connect with those people who are in need of your services right now.

Show them the money

At the risk of using too many *Jerry Maguire* references, sometimes it helps to use math to your advantage. Given that the vast majority of consumers in any market don't need a hospital, health system, or physician at any given time, messages featuring those services will fall on many deaf ears. That can make mass, promotional marketing very ineffective from a cost/benefit standpoint. For hospital non-marketers, this isn't intuitive ("the more we're out there, the better the marketing," right?), and showing them the actual waste involved in old-school hospital marketing can be quite eye-opening (especially for those who value quantitative arguments, such as a CFO).

We created the following calculation based on a real medical center in a real market to help demonstrate just how much waste we're talking about (the organization and market have been hidden to protect the innocent). You can run the numbers on your own to make a similar case.

"Case Study Hospital" (CSH) is regular-sized hospital in a medium-sized market that we'll call Metroville. Now let's say CSH wants to increase its inpatient market share by running a television campaign promoting the awesomeness of the organization's surgeons. (Of course, most new admissions would actually come from physician referrals, past patients, and the emergency department, making this effort even more wasteful—but just play along with us here.) The question is, how many people who see the CSH television campaign will actually be in a position to act upon it?

> Given that the vast majority of consumers in any market don't need a hospital, health system, or physician at any given time, messages featuring those services will fall on many deaf ears.

Over the past year, the CSH service area saw a total of 120,000 surgical inpatient admissions. (Note that we're equating admissions to patients because market share data is typically given as volumes, discharges, or admissions. Given that there are more admissions than unique patients, the targeted numbers are actually smaller than what we're using, making this even more painful. But again, just humor us here.) So that's the target audience, right?

Well, first, we need to cut out those patients who already use CSH—no reason to pay big TV bucks to convince them. CSH has a 13% inpatient share in its service area, or roughly 15,500 patients. That leaves 104,500 potential new patients. (The data we're using is real but would obviously vary depending on the organization, market share, and market size.) Of course, most potential patients are locked into or otherwise loyal to competing hospitals and wouldn't change their care system based on advertising from an alternative. Research we have says that roughly 16% of consumers in a given year are seeking a new hospital, so we'll round that to 15%. Applied to our potential new patient population, that leaves us with 15,675 potential patients who would be seeking a new hospital for surgery in this market.

Stretched out evenly over a year, that equals a targeted audience of roughly 1,300 per month. But let's assume that for every potential patient, there is one other person who might influence our target's healthcare choices (spouse, parent, coworker, etc.) and might be affected by our surgery advertising, so we'll double our targeted audience to 2,600 per month.

Now consider that the television market for CSH is roughly 2.5 million people. The television market of course extends well beyond CSH's primary and secondary service areas, but if we buy a TV spot, that's what we're paying for. Of that audience, we're targeting 2,600 people per month, which means that each month our television advertising and its message of "our surgeons are awesome!" is running, it will be relevant to roughly 2,600 out of 2.5 million folks, or 1 out of every 1,000 people. That is some seriously ineffective "targeted" marketing. We are using the most expensive marketing technique available to reach a scant 2,600 people who are in a position to consider our services. In addition, that massive expense is virtually wasted on 2,497,400 others who have no need for surgery or are far beyond our service area. All we can hope for is some awareness or perceptions boost, which will be severely limited both by the fact that our message is irrelevant to that audience and because any impact typically lasts only while the advertising is in the market, and perhaps for a short time afterward.

Put another way—those people who will find your surgery-focused messaging relevant are like a rare fish found in the Atlantic Ocean. Mass advertising is the equivalent of building a net the length of the Atlantic seaboard and dragging the ocean for that rare fish. Very expensive and very ineffective. Digital and content marketing using relevant messages and channels is like finding out what kind of food that fish really loves, dropping that bait in targeted areas, and waiting for the fish to come to you.

Remember the core principles of change management

There are some common strategies for managing organizational change that apply to marketers wanting to shift to the new paradigm. A great resource for change management is John Kotter's *The Heart of Change*, but here are some relevant common principles:

Create a burning platform—Those who resist change ("everyone has a billboard!" "we need to tell our story!" "we need revenue—we need to get on TV!") often need to hear a compelling "why" regarding change, and many experts advocate building the "why" around the fear of what happens if you don't change. Given the shift in healthcare consumers and how they engage brands, the rise of accessible information and transparency, mobile and social media, and reform, there is plenty of fodder for building the case that healthcare organizations that don't change their marketing approach will fall behind their competitors in terms of effectiveness and efficiency in marketing.

Communicate early and often—You may need to make your sales pitch for moving away from the old paradigm to the new many times over. Given that it will likely be a new strategy to many non-marketers, don't assume that one email or presentation will pave the way. You will likely have to defend your efforts multiple times over. Knowing this, look for ongoing opportunities to make your case—at board sessions, leadership meetings, one-on-one conversations, official internal communications, and more. And be sure to look for influential members outside of your marketing department who can serve as champions for your efforts along the way. Best-case scenario, start laying the groundwork for the new approach well before you begin, allowing your internal audiences more time to wrestle with and accept what may be a very foreign concept. When you do start to build enthusiasm and support from leadership, it's critical to keep that momentum going—they'll easily forget otherwise.

> If moving toward new, transformational marketing efforts were easy, the logical case would be enough.

Create a pilot effort and celebrate early success—In a paper I wrote on patient experience innovation in 2007, I advocated using the "iPod Mind-set." One of the main tenets of this philosophy is to think small with change. That is, instead of trying to completely overhaul your marketing strategies, which might frighten those in your organization who aren't ready for sweeping change, build a pilot effort. For example, create a content marketing program for one service line, which will allow you to continue the traditional efforts that make everyone comfortable while you build a success story that can more quickly (and with less disruption) demonstrate the efficacy of your strategy.

If moving toward new, transformational marketing efforts were easy, the logical case would be enough. But any form of true transformation must reach beyond the logical to the personal, the emotional, and the irrational. That's what change management is all about, and the more you can wrap your content marketing program into change management strategies, the more success you are likely to have.

• • •

IN CLOSING

In *Joe Public Doesn't Care About Your Hospital*, I closed with "The Healthcare Marketer's Oath," a call to marketers to commit to the changes outlined in that book. It was one of the only clear calls to action in the book, which was intentionally designed as a manifesto to argue change in a slow-moving, often antiquated healthcare marketing industry. In this book, the calls to action are many and crystal clear, and my hope is that this book will serve as your guide to break through to the other side.

For sure, this book provides a high-level framework and is really only the start in terms of what you will need to learn and understand. With that said, I have attempted to provide you—at both the strategic and tactical level—with a clear path for moving out of the existing old-school marketing paradigm based on promotional mass advertising into the new paradigm that emphasizes digital and content marketing. Not only should the philosophies you need to embrace be clear, but the benchmarks to measure your progress should be obvious as well. You have read what it takes to develop the digital marketing mind-set; master digital channels, tools, and resources; and understand the four attributes of digital marketing mastery. You have learned the value of content marketing and what it means to go vertical with your content marketing programs. You have seen workable strategies for preparing your organization for the tough changes ahead. You have read about those healthcare marketers who have blazed the trail ahead of you, who have finally crossed the great divide into the new paradigm. They have found enlightenment, professional achievement, and marketing success there. Remember the story in the introduction in which the marketing team was poised to move boldly into the new paradigm and recognized the challenge with a "holy &%$#" moment? Just before this book went to press, I received this message from the marketing leader:

> "Hi Chris! I wanted to give you an update and great news. We have been touring around the organization, presenting our new campaign to key leadership groups. Today we had what has traditionally been our toughest audience: physician leaders. In past meetings with them, they have been VERY vocal and unhappy about our marketing efforts.
>
> Today there was a change. They were very enthusiastically supportive of our campaign. During the section about content marketing, one of the most vocal physicians spoke up about his support for the concept. I think the fact that it is differentiating from our competition really resonated with him and the others.
>
> There are more efforts in the works—we are really making progress!"

The path was not easy for them, nor will it be for you. But you are now armed and ready to join them. You have the tools, you have the map, you have the faith. You are ready to make the leap into the new paradigm.

Now, what are you waiting for?

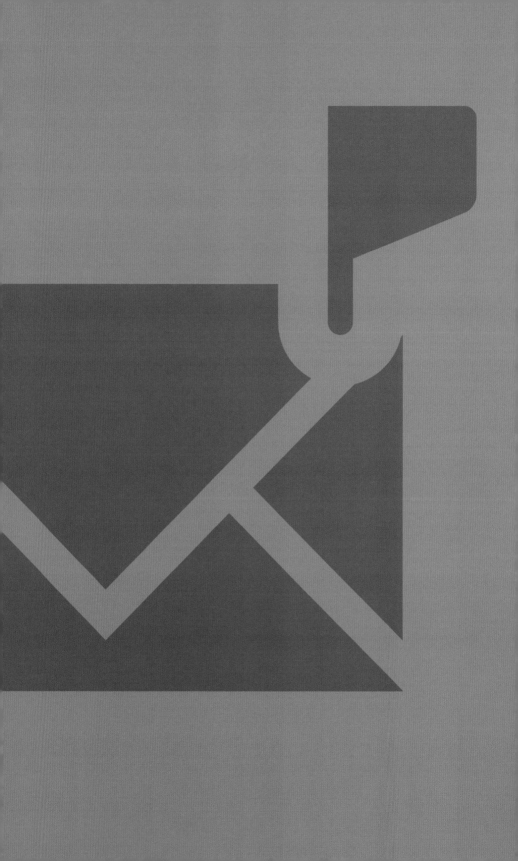

HOW TO
STAY CONNECTED

Want to learn more about how to move to the new consumer health-care marketing paradigm? Take advantage of these resources:

Reach out to author Chris Bevolo directly at chris@thinkinterval.com or follow him on Twitter at @IntervalChris.

Learn how Interval helps healthcare organizations move into the new paradigm with services focused on digital strategy, content marketing, and interactive design, and explore our cache of content including articles, papers, videos, webinars, and more.

Visit thinkinterval.com

Subscribe to ongoing content from Interval on digital marketing, content marketing, and more.

Visit thinkinterval.com/subscribe

Listen to Interval's weekly podcast, the Arrogant Healthcare Marketing Bastards, as we discuss healthcare marketing trends, topics, and ideas (with some other fun stuff thrown in).

Visit thinkinterval.com/ahmb or subscribe on iTunes.

Register for an upcoming Joe Public Retreats, an intense, two-day experience to learn more on how to master digital marketing, content marketing, or other strategic marketing practices.

Visit joepublicretreat.com

Don't forget to visit IntervalAudit.com for a free online digital marketing audit.

ENDNOTES

1. Chris Bevolo, *A Marketer's Guide to Measuring Results: Prove the Impact of New Media and Traditional Healthcare Marketing Efforts* (Marblehead MA: HCPro, 2010), 53.

2. Robert Hof, "Google Research: No mobile site = lost customers," *Forbes.com*, September 25, 2012, http://www.forbes.com/sites/roberthof/2012/09/25/google-research-no-mobile-site-lost-customers/

3. "The Digital Journey to Wellness: Hospital Selection," thinkwithgoogle.com, September 2012, http://www.thinkwithgoogle.com/research-studies/the-digital-journey-to-wellness-hospital-selection.html

4. Marty Neumeier, *The Brand Gap: How to Bridge the Distance Between Business Strategy and Design* (Indianapolis: New Riders, 2003), 2–3.

5. David Marlowe, *A Marketer's Guide to Measuring ROI: Tools to Track the Returns From Healthcare Marketing Efforts* (Marblehead MA: HCPro, 2007)

6. Peter Achinstein, *Science Rules: A Historical Introduction to Scientific Methods* (Baltimore, MD: The Johns Hopkins University Press, August 2004), 358.

7. Wikipedia.com, http://en.wikipedia.org/wiki/Giordano_Bruno